MY HOSPITAL ADVENTURE

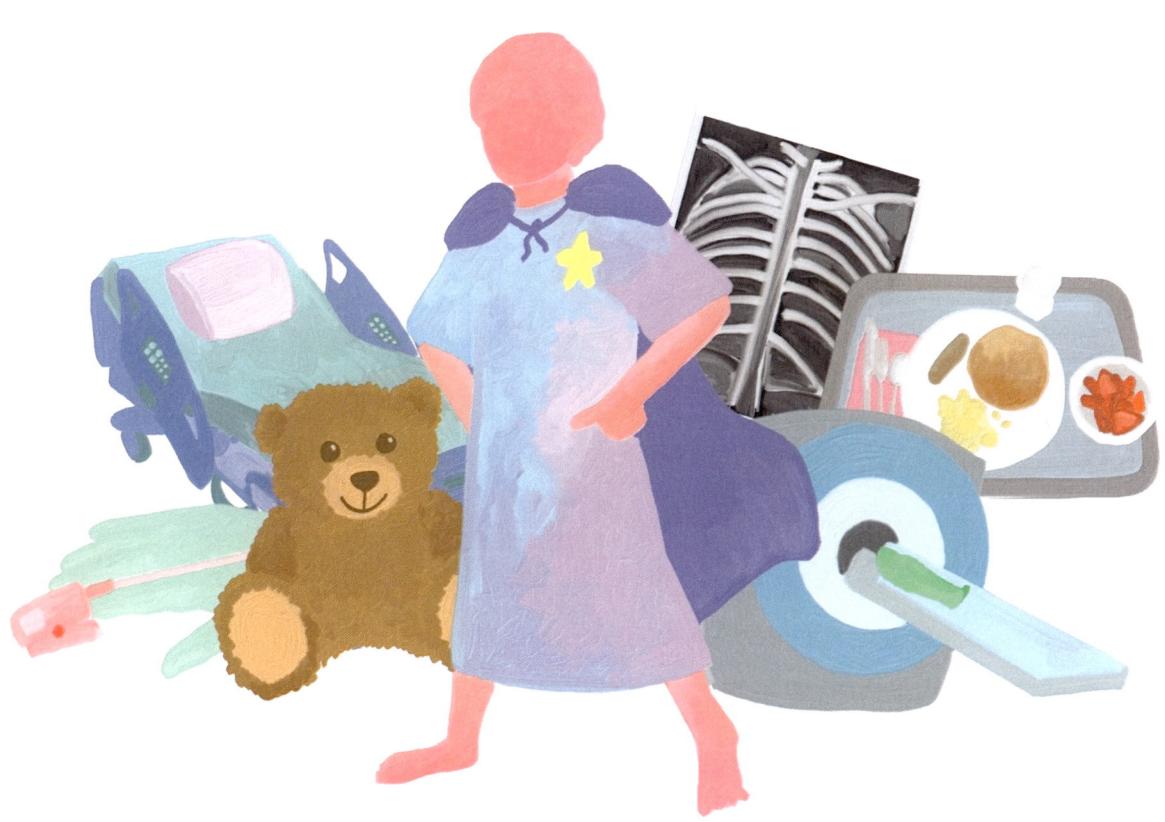

Commissioned by
The Blank Children's Hospital
Child Life Department

Written and Illustrated by
Laura Camerona, CCLS
at

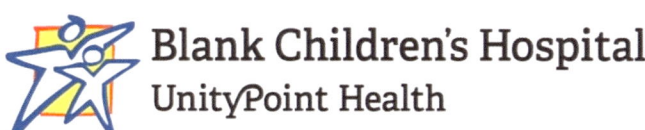

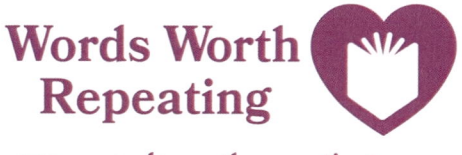

www.wordsworthrepeating.com

Notes for Adults Reading This Book with a Child Before, During, or After a Hospital Stay

Each child needs different things. Before experiencing something stressful, some kids do better when they get information that helps them understand and helps them know what to expect. Other children do better not thinking about it a lot. These children may benefit from processing after. In general, caregivers know their children the best. So please use this book as you see fit.

The book has a main storyline that is appropriate for younger children. It is suggested you start there. If your child has more questions or can handle more information, there are prompts to help a child discuss their own experiences and lots of additional information on the bottom of each page. In addition, there is a fun and educational Hospital Adventure Guide in the back of the book. This portion of the book is meant to be used as a reference. There are interactive activities and tools to help families find what works best for their child. Most children will not need all of the information in this guide. Share what you think would be helpful to your child.

Lastly, there is help beyond the words in the book. If your child is needing further support, medical professionals can help your family before, during, or after a hospitalization. Ask your medical team to refer you to a Child Life Specialist or a social worker/therapist who is familiar with medical treatment and coping.

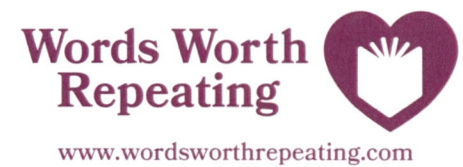

Words Worth Repeating

www.wordsworthrepeating.com

Des Moines, Iowa

I am a brave explorer,
and I have just returned
from a big adventure!

I spent the night at the hospital.

I met new people. I tried new
things. I did stuff that I had
never done before.

It was like exploring
a whole new world!

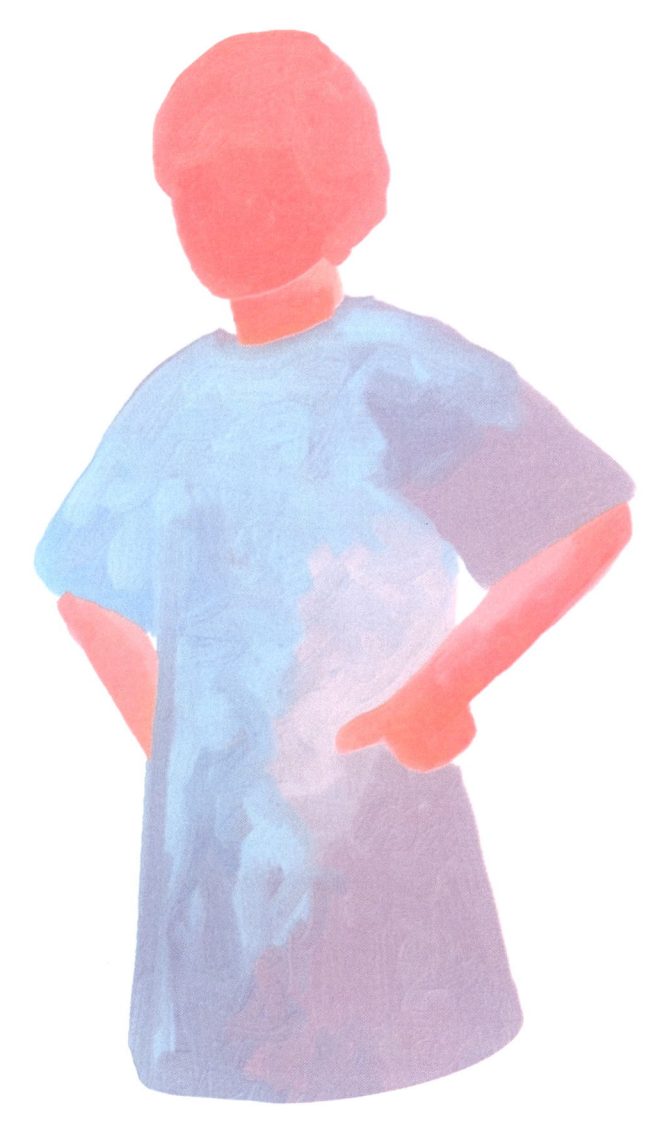

What do you think brave looks like?

Brave can be different for different people.
Brave means that you have courage.
Brave means that you are ready to face new things.
Brave means trying to find the best way to go through something hard.
A brave person can still cry. A brave person can still tell someone
when something doesn't feel good.

I saw a lot of new things, and sometimes, it even seemed like the people I met were speaking a different language. I'm so excited to tell you all about it!

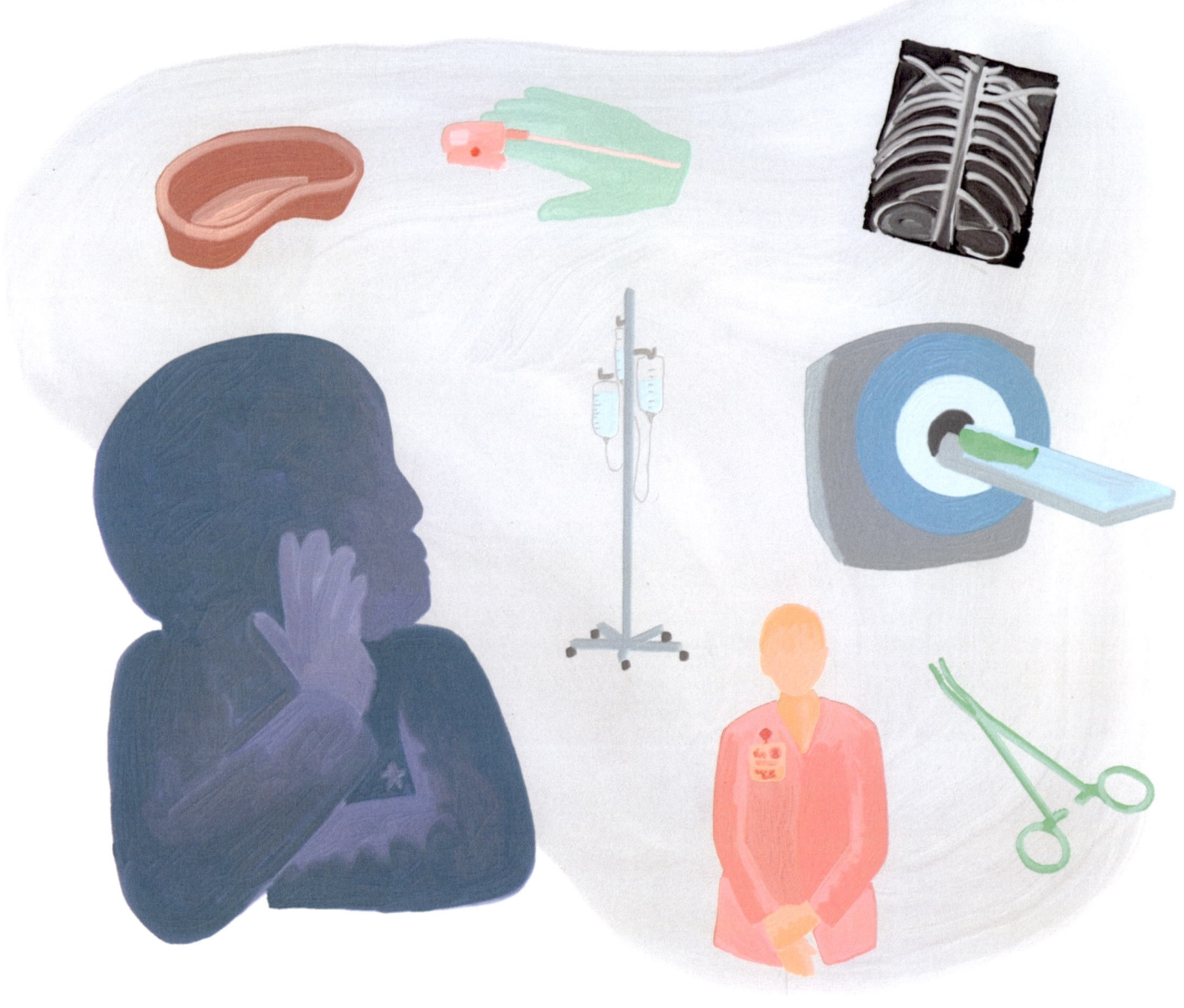

Words can have different meanings in the hospital. This can be confusing. If someone explains something in words you don't understand, it is okay to ask them to explain it in a different way.

Admitted: When a person is checked into the hospital to spend the night.

Patient: A person who a doctor takes care of.

At the hospital, I had my very own room with a special bed. The bed could move up and down, and I could push a button to make it sit up. I liked to pretend it was my very own spaceship.

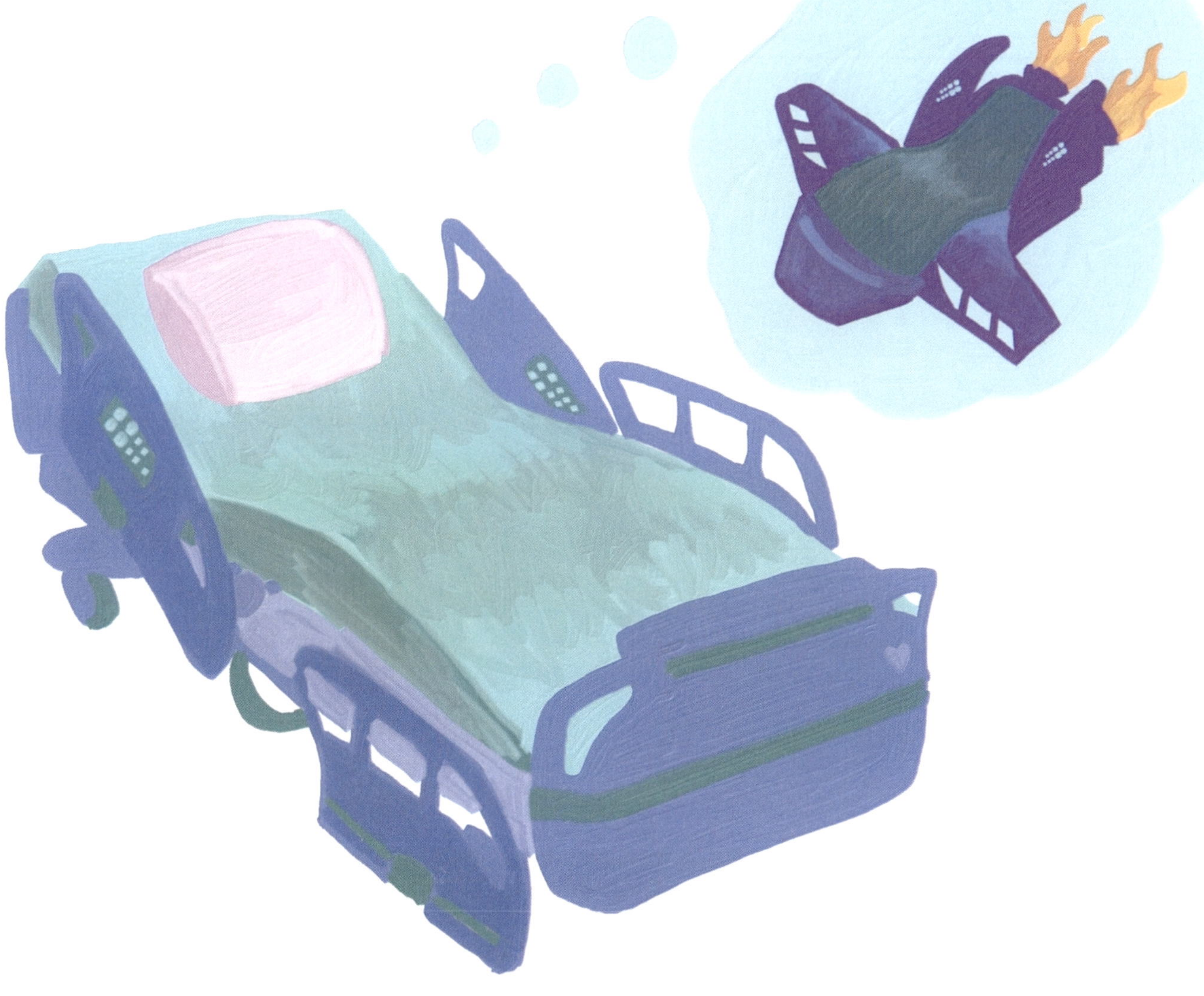

Call Light: Each hospital room has a special button that can be used to call the nurse. When you push the special button, a light outside of the room shines so the nurse knows that you need to be checked on.

In the hospital, your grown-up can stay in your room with you. They might sleep on the couch, chair, or extra bed in the room. The hospital also has cribs for babies and young children.

What else could you pretend your hospital bed is?

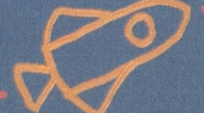

Lots of people wore clothes that were a little different than what I am used to. I wore hospital pajamas and a special bracelet with my name on it.

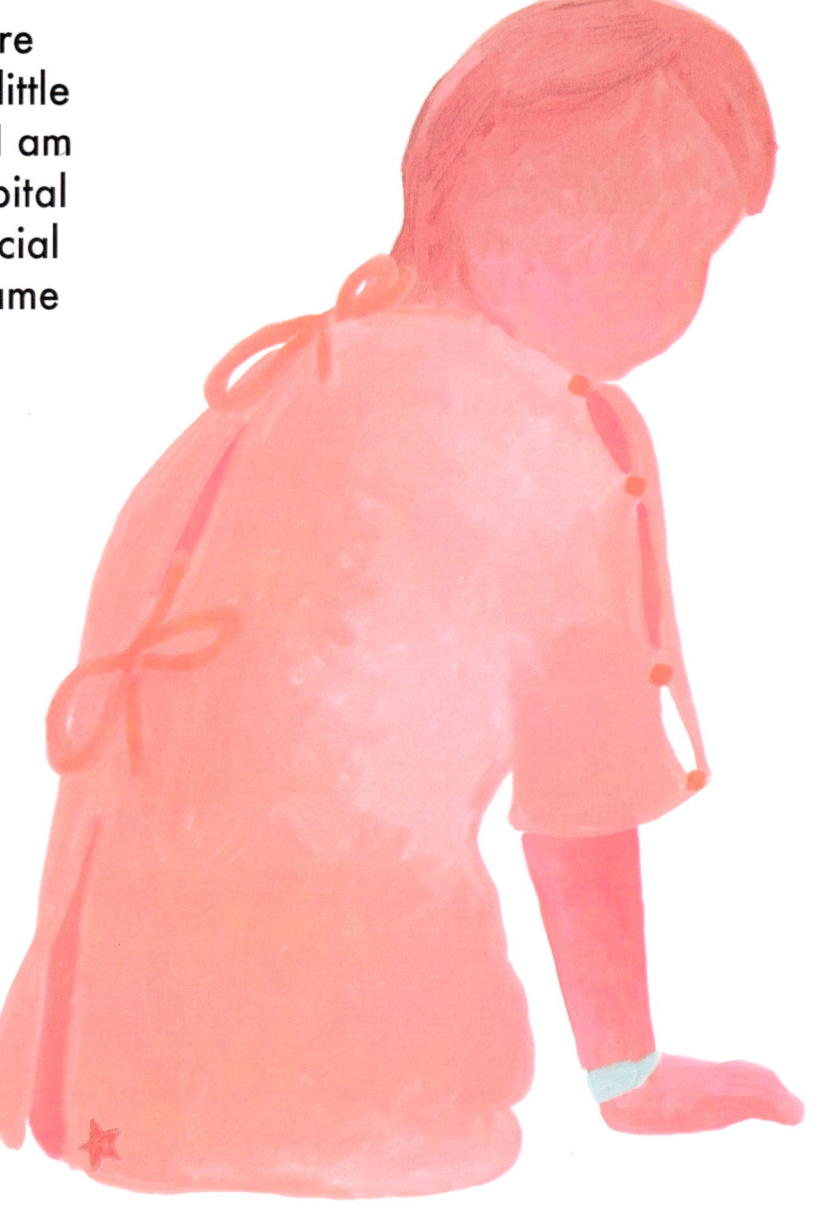

The snaps and ties on hospital pajamas make it easier for nurses to check parts of your body. Hospital pajamas are also easier to take on and off when you are laying down or if things are connected to your body.

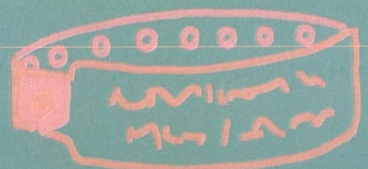

Hospital bracelets are important because they can help nurses quickly check that they have the right person before they give them medicine or help them in some way. A nurse might use a scanner to 'beep' your bracelet. Some kids thinks it sounds like the grocery store check out!

The people who worked at the hospital wore special clothes called scrubs. I thought the scrubs looked like they were wearing pajamas like me.

My adventure was a one big pajama party!

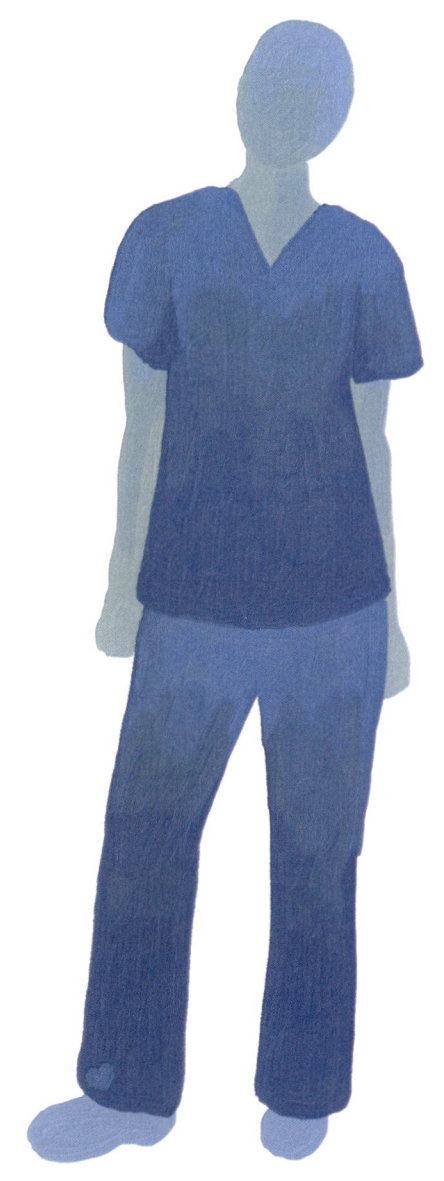

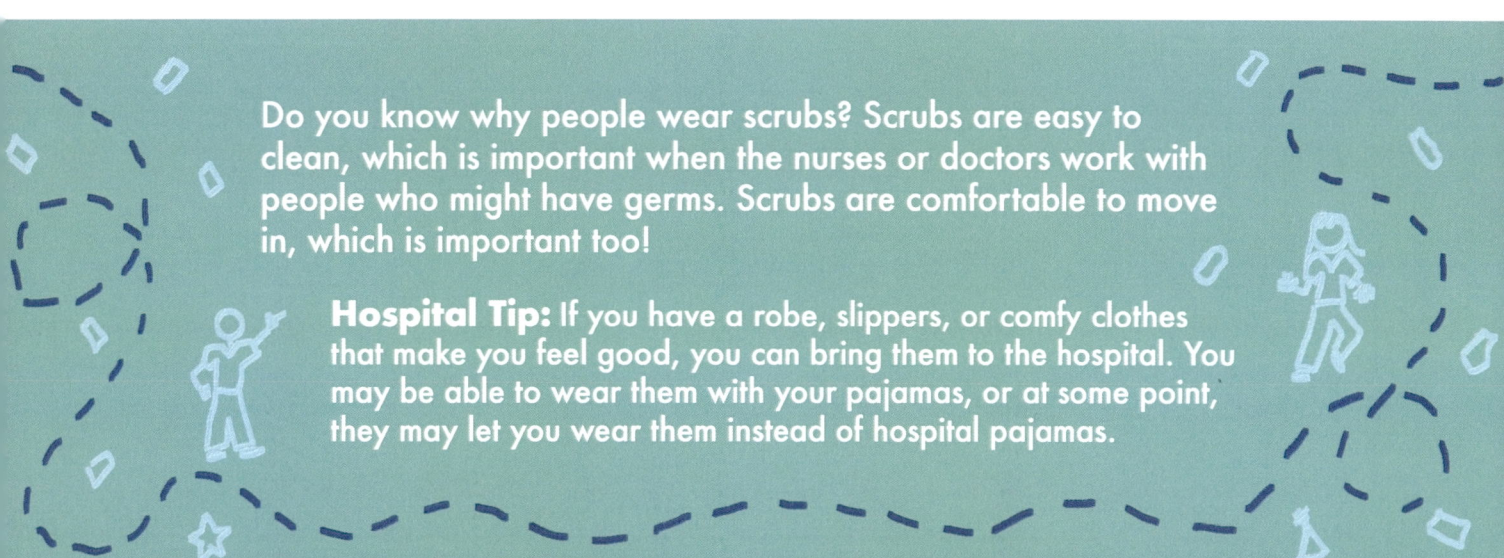

Do you know why people wear scrubs? Scrubs are easy to clean, which is important when the nurses or doctors work with people who might have germs. Scrubs are comfortable to move in, which is important too!

Hospital Tip: If you have a robe, slippers, or comfy clothes that make you feel good, you can bring them to the hospital. You may be able to wear them with your pajamas, or at some point, they may let you wear them instead of hospital pajamas.

Some people at the hospital wore masks. The masks were important because they kept people from catching other people's germs.

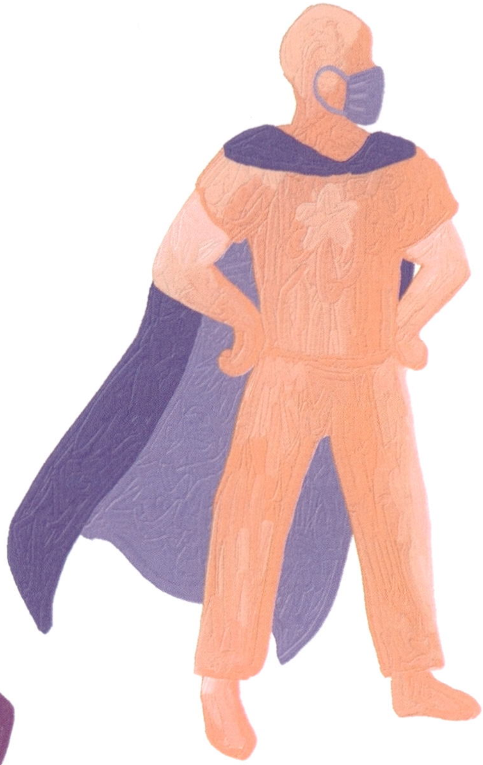

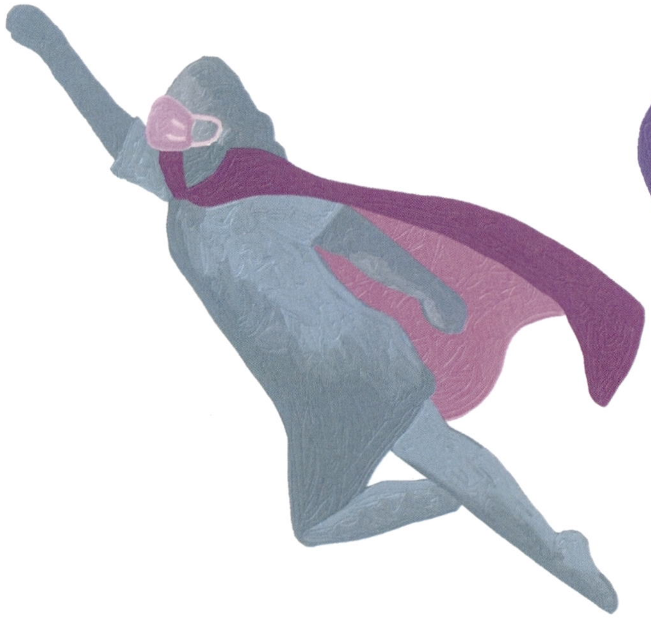

Sometimes, I had to wear a mask too.
I liked to call it my superhero mask!

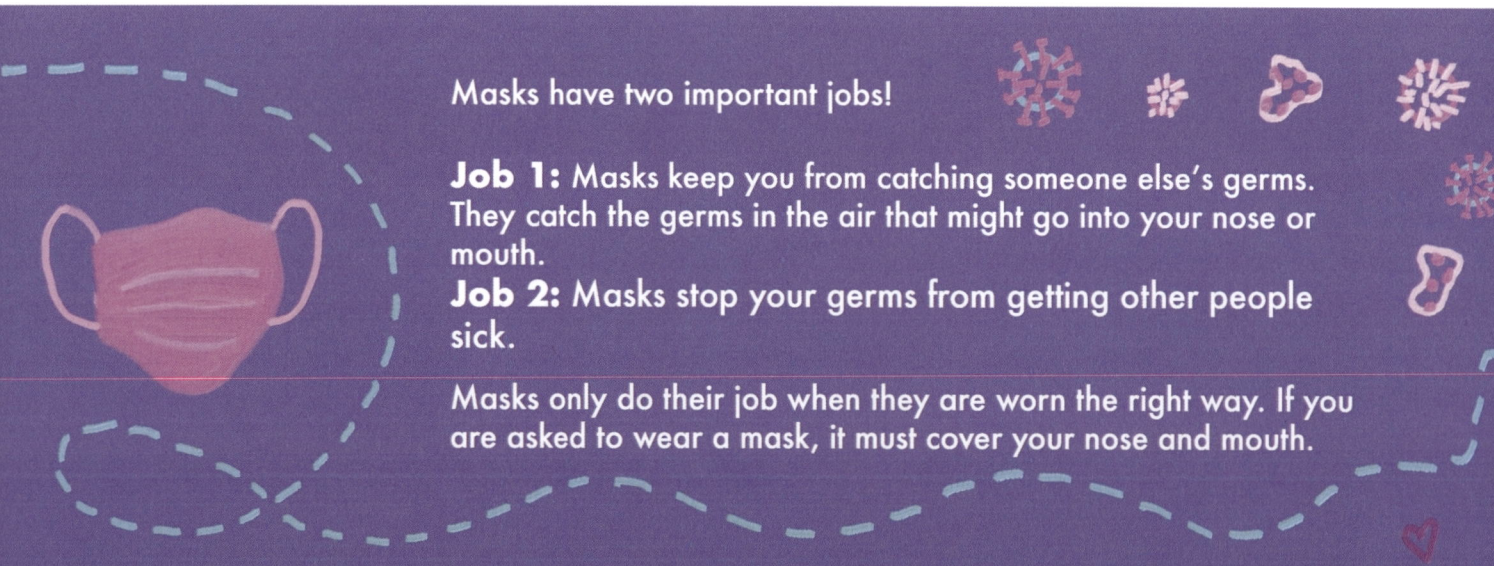

Masks have two important jobs!

Job 1: Masks keep you from catching someone else's germs. They catch the germs in the air that might go into your nose or mouth.

Job 2: Masks stop your germs from getting other people sick.

Masks only do their job when they are worn the right way. If you are asked to wear a mask, it must cover your nose and mouth.

I met so many people on my adventure. There are people at the hospital with so many different jobs. It was fun to learn about what everyone does.

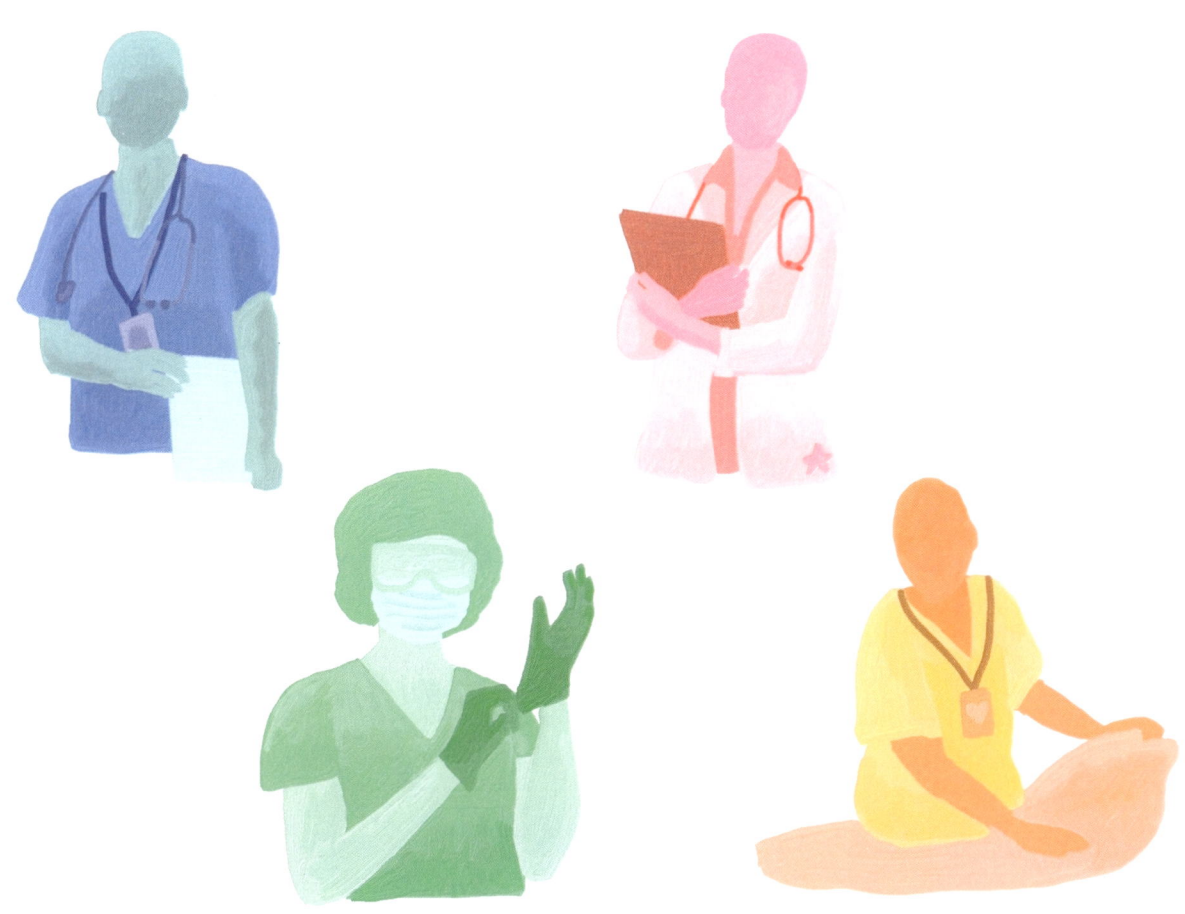

When I met new people, I also liked to ask them what their favorite animal was. When I am on an adventure, I like to find ways to have fun!

If you are in the mood to be a little silly, you could ask everyone you meet the same question and keep track of their answers. For example, what's your favorite...
...Food from the cafeteria?
...Place to travel? ...Color?
...Cartoon? ...Cereal?

There is a cool page in the Adventure Guide where you can check off the people you meet and write down their answers to your silly question!

Laughter is so good for the body! When you laugh, your body creates more cells that fight germs. Laughing can also make your brain send signals that help your body feel less pain and stress.

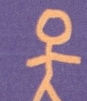

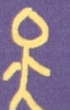
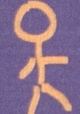
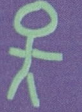
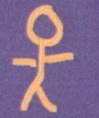
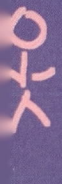
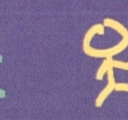
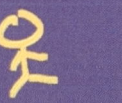

A lot of the people asked me the same questions over and over. This got a little old, but sometimes, when you are on an adventure, you have to do things that are a little annoying.

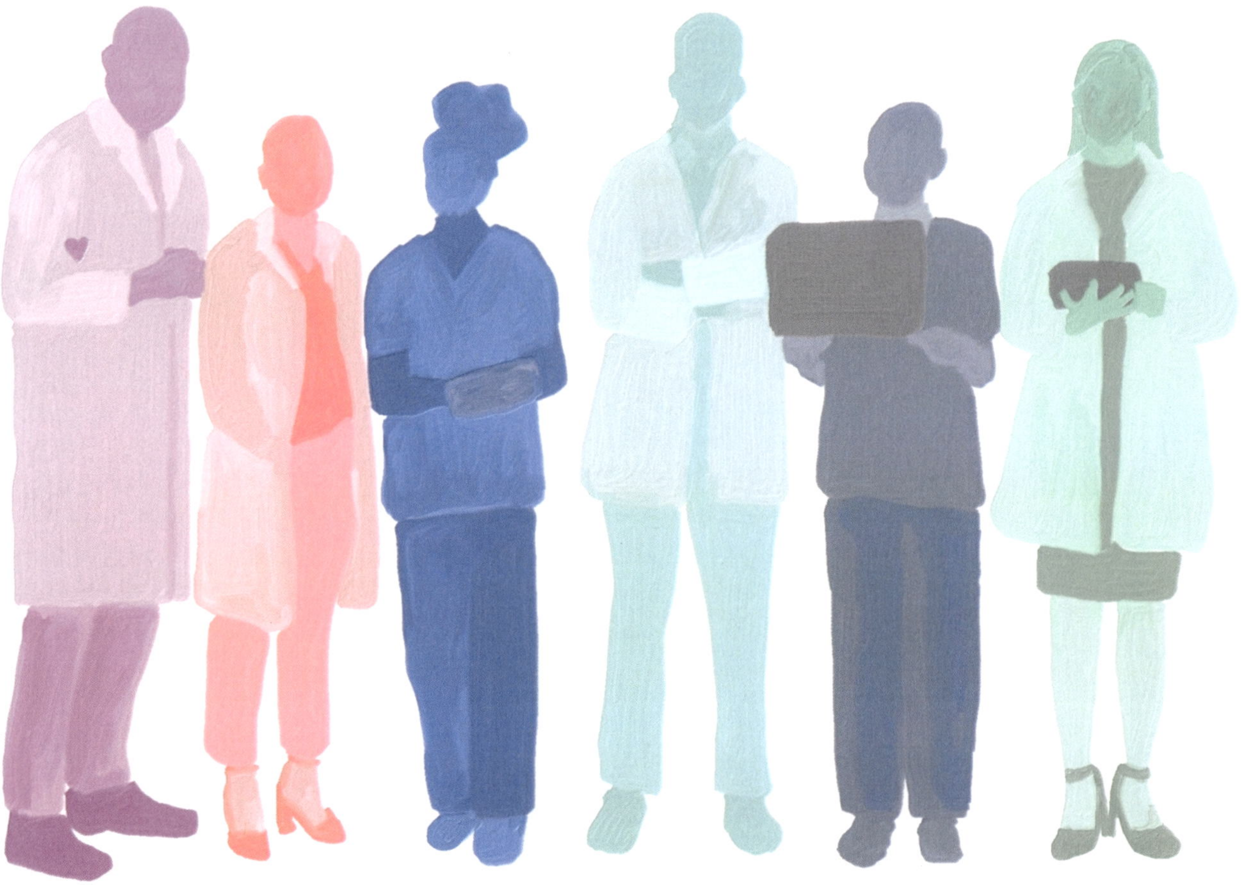

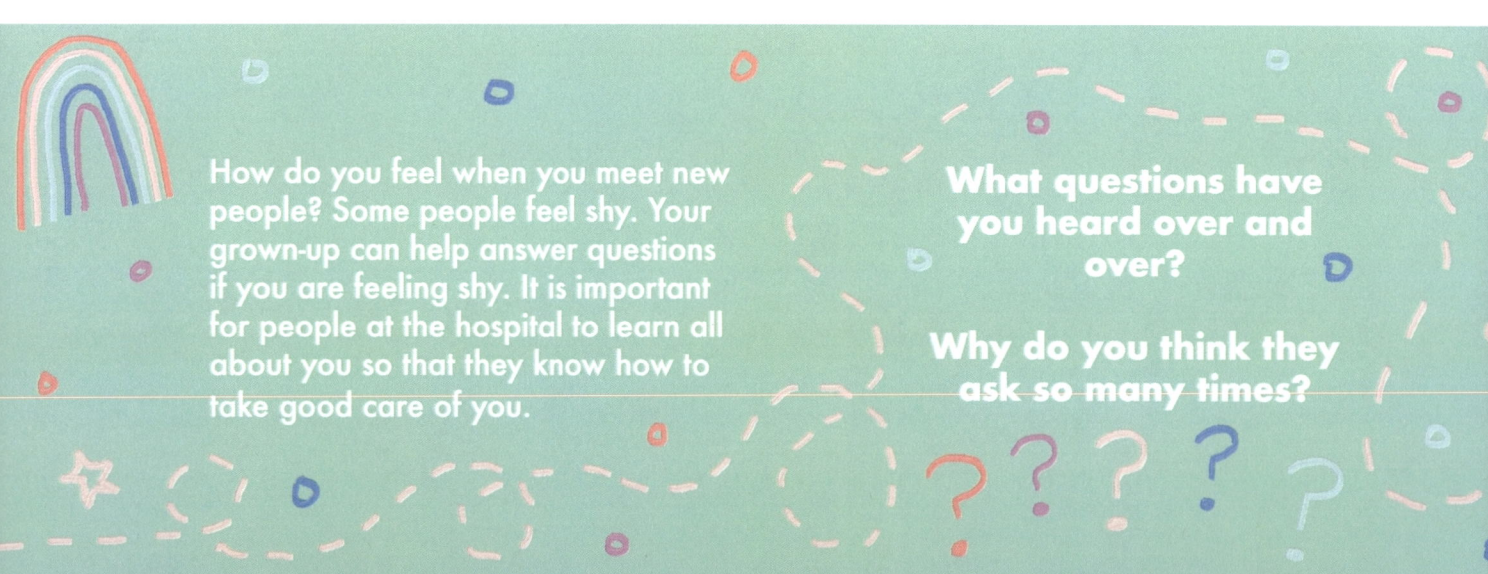

How do you feel when you meet new people? Some people feel shy. Your grown-up can help answer questions if you are feeling shy. It is important for people at the hospital to learn all about you so that they know how to take good care of you.

What questions have you heard over and over?

Why do you think they ask so many times?

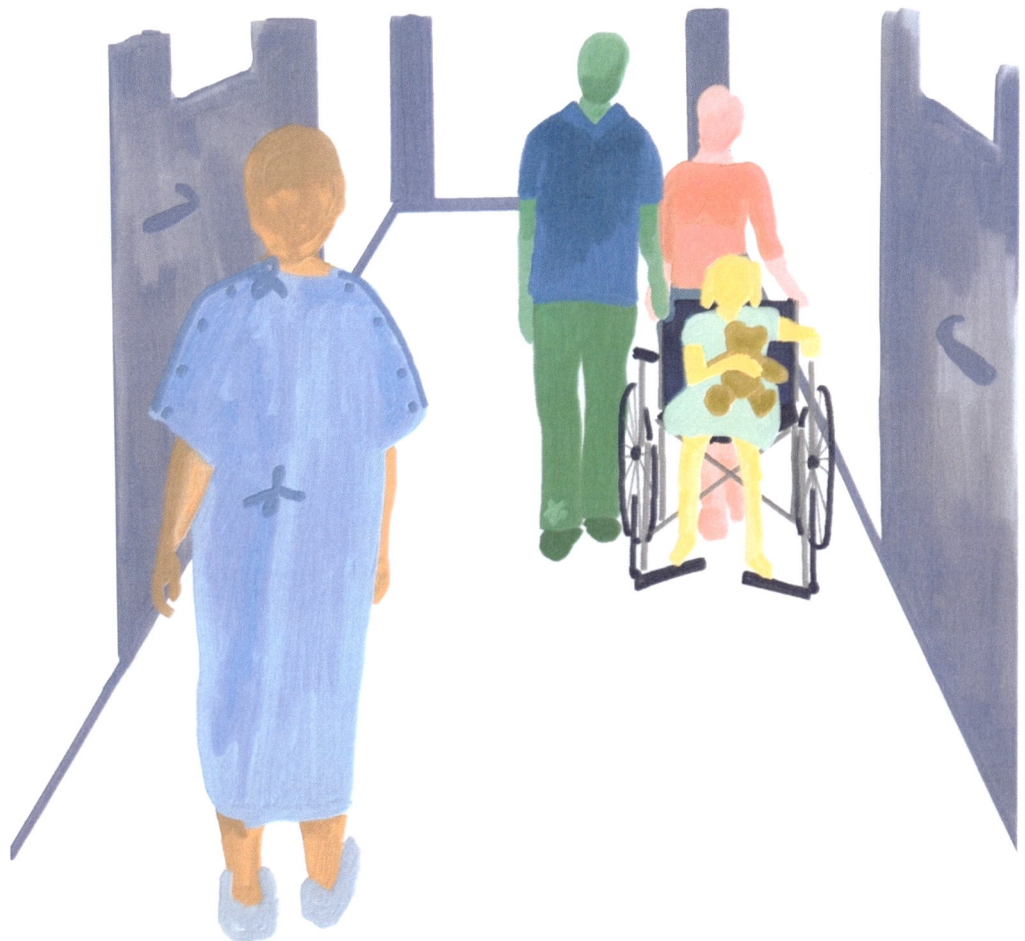

There were other kids at the hospital too, but I didn't see them much because I had my very own room. It was nice to know that other kids were doing the same things that I was. Sometimes, I would see another kid in the hall wearing hospital pajamas too.

Sometimes, people in the hospital share a room or stay in an extra space until a room is ready for them. The people at the hospital will still work to get them everything they need and to give them privacy.

Hospital Tip: The hospital has pillows and blankets, but if it helps you sleep, you can bring your favorite pillow or stuffed animal from home. You could also bring pictures, a book, or a movie that makes you feel good.

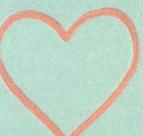
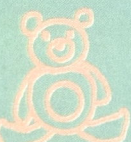

When someone goes on a hospital adventure, it means their body needs special care that they can't get at home. People stay at the hospital for different reasons.
Everyone's adventure is different.

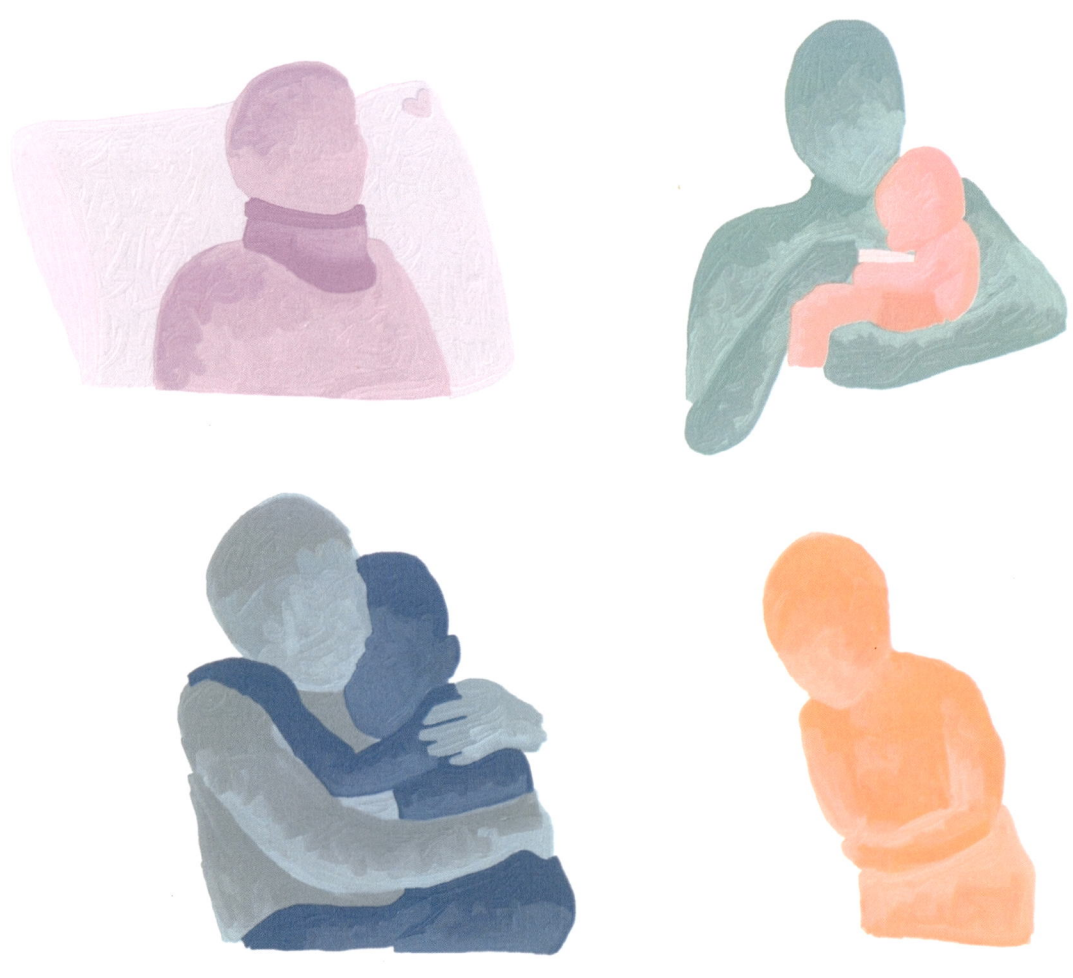

You can learn more about the different parts of your body that might need help in the Hospital Adventure Guide at the end of this book.

Kids come to the hospital in different ways. Some kids go to the emergency room first. Many kids are brought to the hospital by their grown-up.

In an emergency, some kids come to the hospital in an ambulance or helicopter!

How have you traveled to the hospital?

Part of my hospital adventure was working with the doctors and nurses to figure out what was going on and what would help my body the most. The doctors looked at my throat, nose, and ears and listened to my breathing.

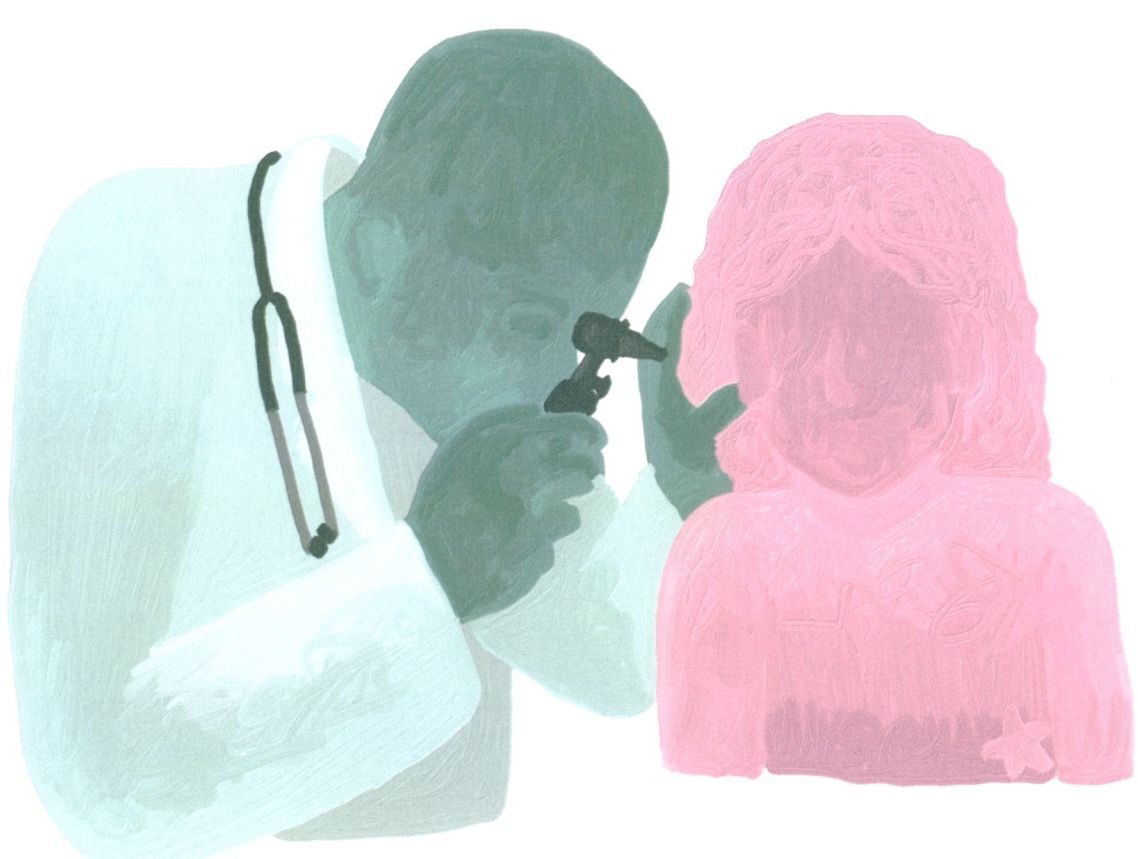

Here are a few more words that have different meanings at the hospital:

○ ○ ○ ○ ○ ○ ○

Test: In the hospital, it DOES NOT mean that you have to take a test!
A test at the hospital is when a doctor checks out a certain part of a person's body to see how it is working.

Lab: In the hospital, it DOES NOT mean a kind of dog. The lab is a place with different kinds of microscopes and machines that count cells, look for germs, and learn more about how someone's body is working.

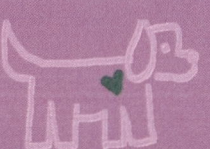
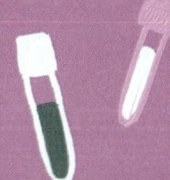

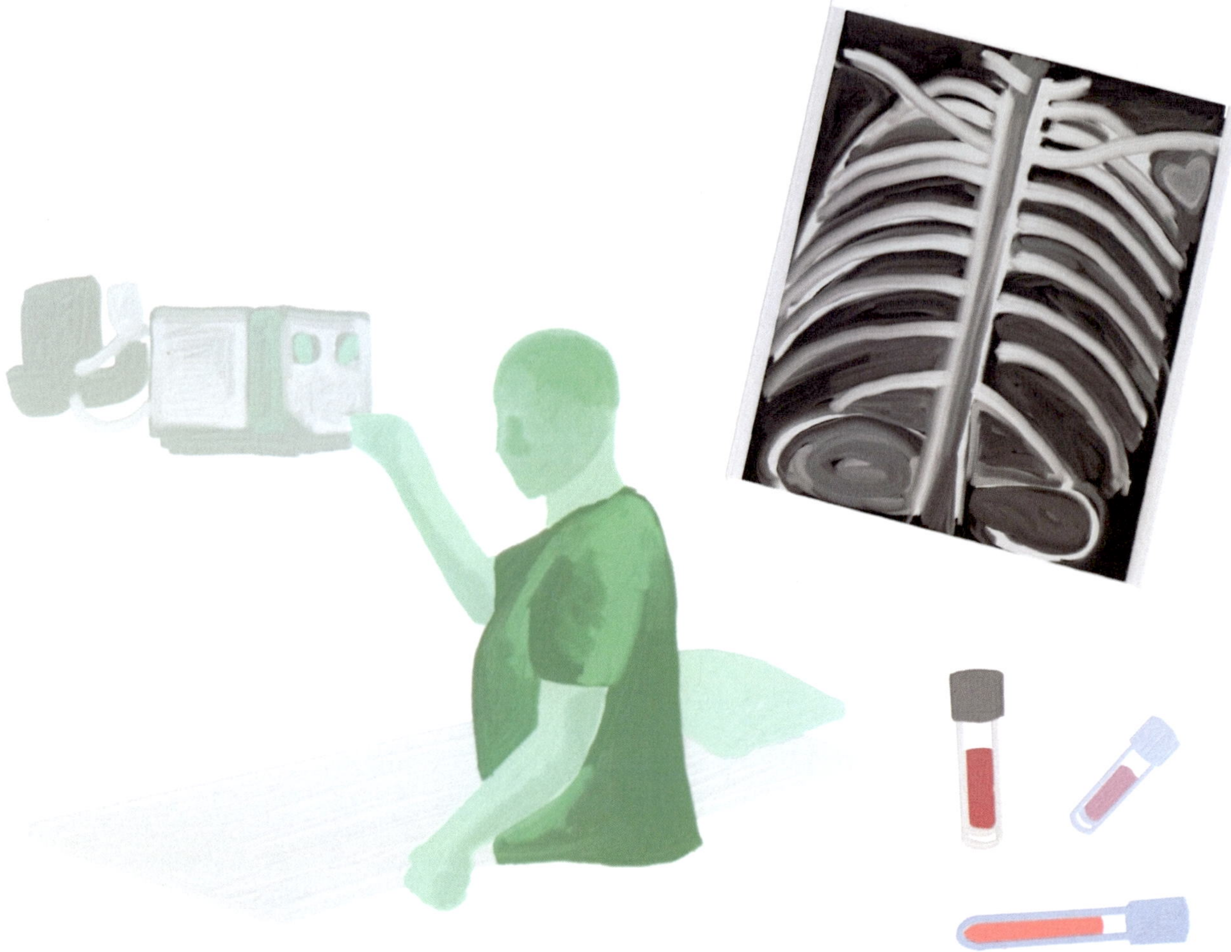

During my adventure, the hospital used a special camera to take pictures of the inside of my body. The hospital sent a little bit of my blood to a place called a lab, where someone could look at it closely. There are lots of ways to learn about what is going on inside of a body.

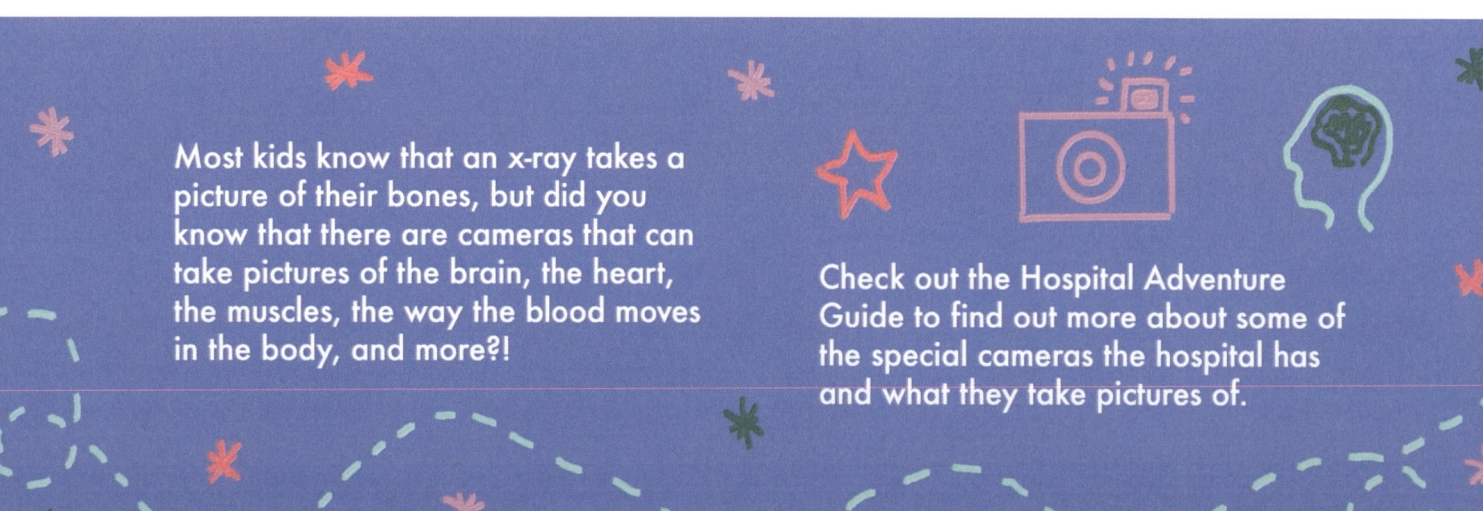

Most kids know that an x-ray takes a picture of their bones, but did you know that there are cameras that can take pictures of the brain, the heart, the muscles, the way the blood moves in the body, and more?!

Check out the Hospital Adventure Guide to find out more about some of the special cameras the hospital has and what they take pictures of.

When I was at the hospital, the nurses would check my temperature, my heart, and my breathing every few hours.

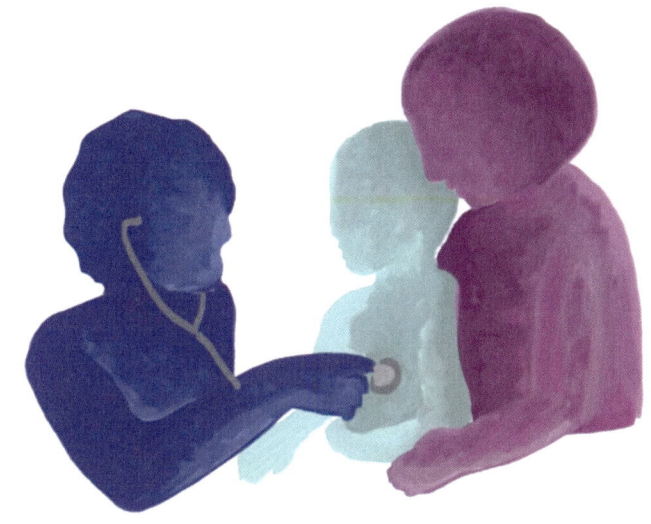

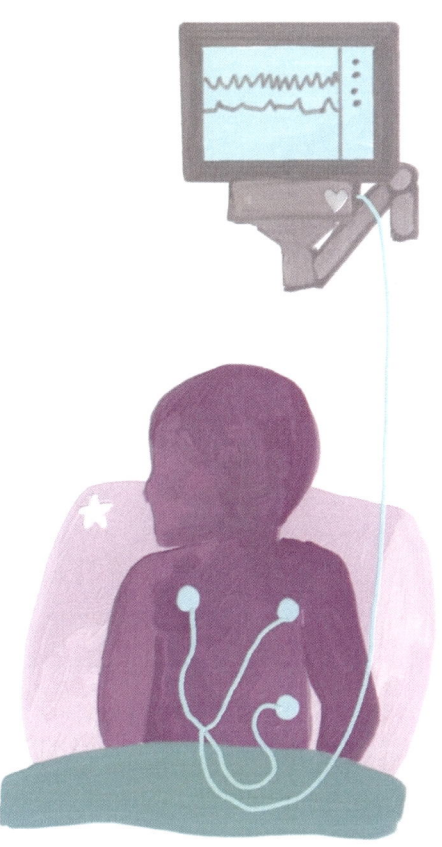

The hospital had some really cool tools that helped. The nurses used a stethoscope, some special stickers, and a little red light. None of these things hurt at all!

Stethoscope: A tool that can be used to listen to someone's heartbeat and the sounds that the lungs make when they breathe.

PulseOx: The "little red light" that senses how much oxygen is in someone's blood. The light shines through someone's finger or toe and the sensor on the other side can tell how much oxygen got in the way of the light.

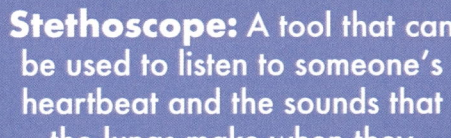

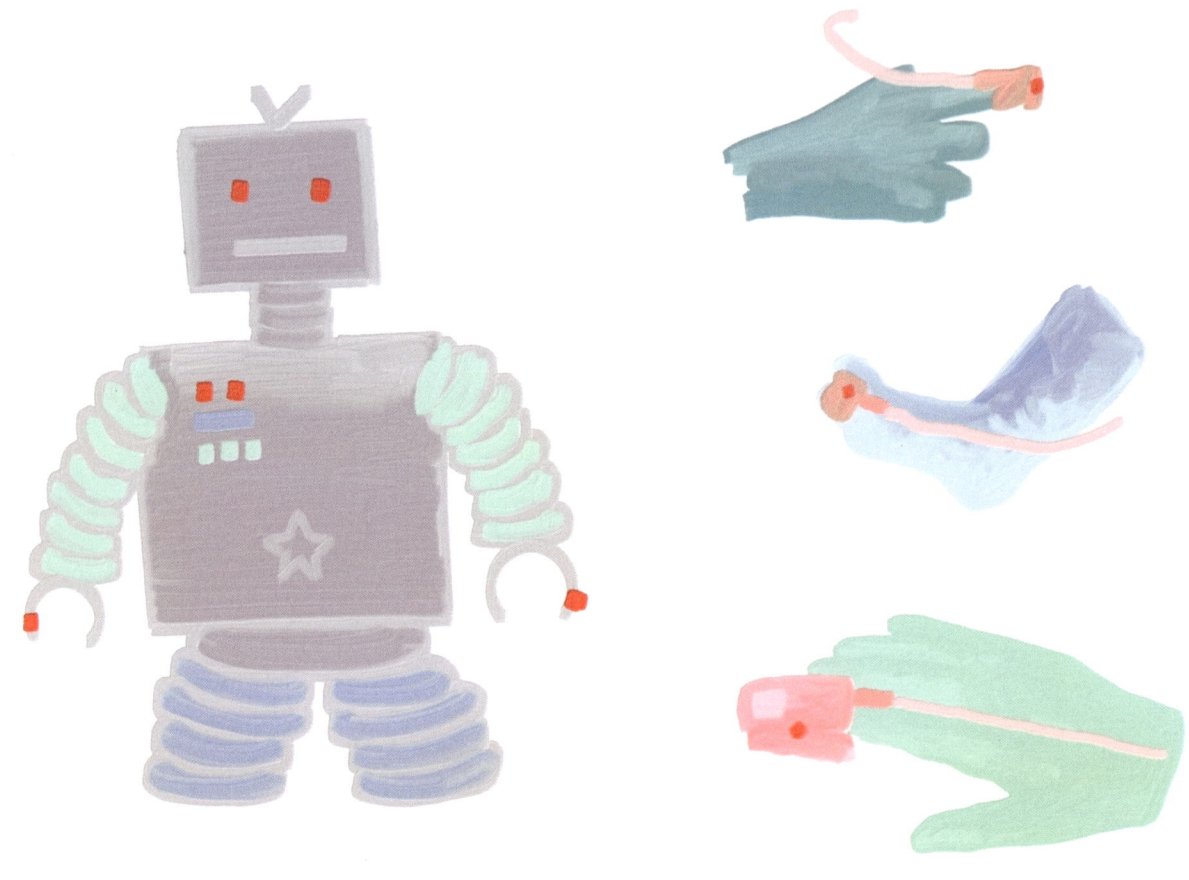

The stickers and the red light could send a message about my heart and my breathing to a computer in my room.
It was super cool. I liked to pretend that I was a robot!

Vitals: When a nurse comes into the room to check how fast your heart is beating, your temperature, and your breathing, this is called "checking your vitals."

Oxygen: When we breathe in air, our body pulls oxygen out of the air. Our body sends the oxygen all over our body through the blood stream.

Learn more about oxygen, the lungs, and the heart in the Hospital Adventure Guide!

 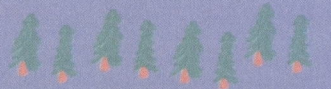 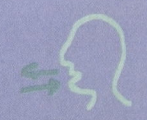

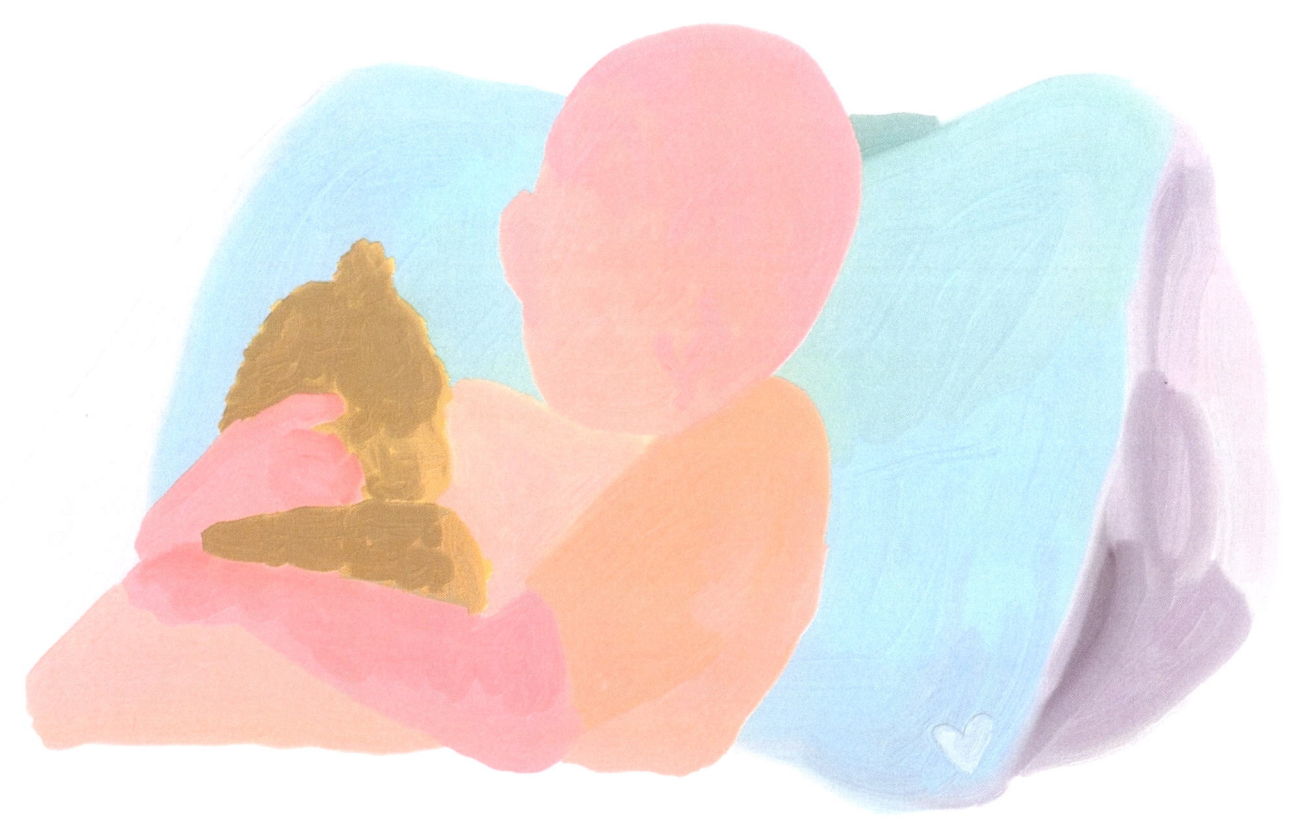

Every brave explorer has a mission.

My mission during my hospital adventure was to work with
my doctors and nurses to get my body healthy
so that I could go back home.

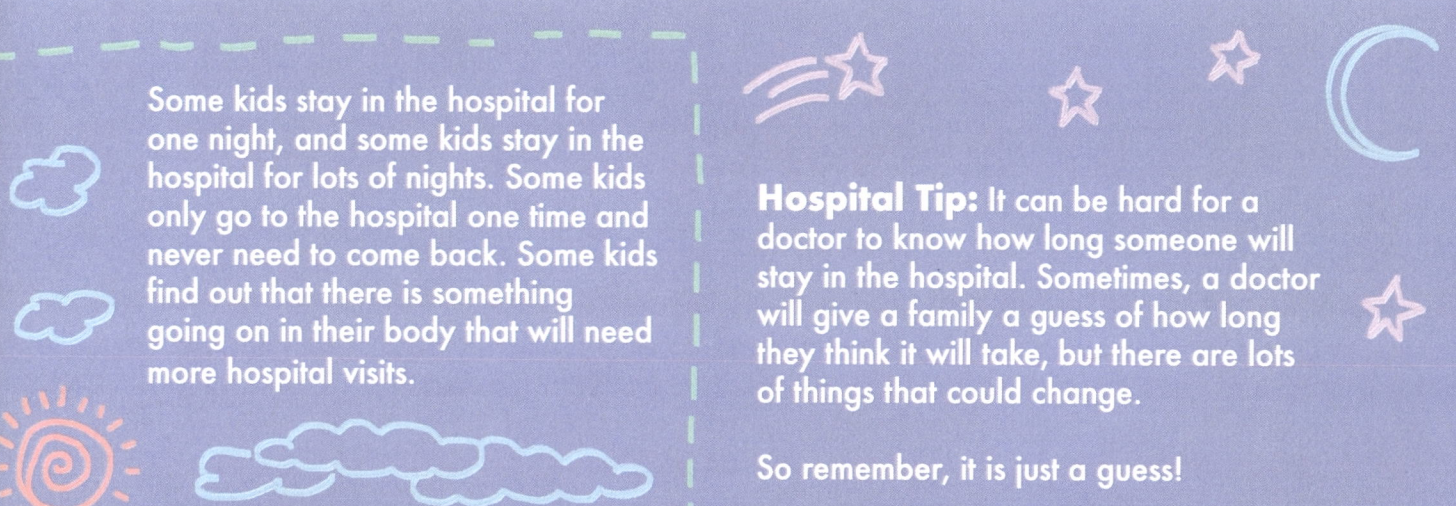

Some kids stay in the hospital for one night, and some kids stay in the hospital for lots of nights. Some kids only go to the hospital one time and never need to come back. Some kids find out that there is something going on in their body that will need more hospital visits.

Hospital Tip: It can be hard for a doctor to know how long someone will stay in the hospital. Sometimes, a doctor will give a family a guess of how long they think it will take, but there are lots of things that could change.

So remember, it is just a guess!

Luckily, I had my grown-up as a sidekick! A sidekick is someone who helps an explorer with their mission.

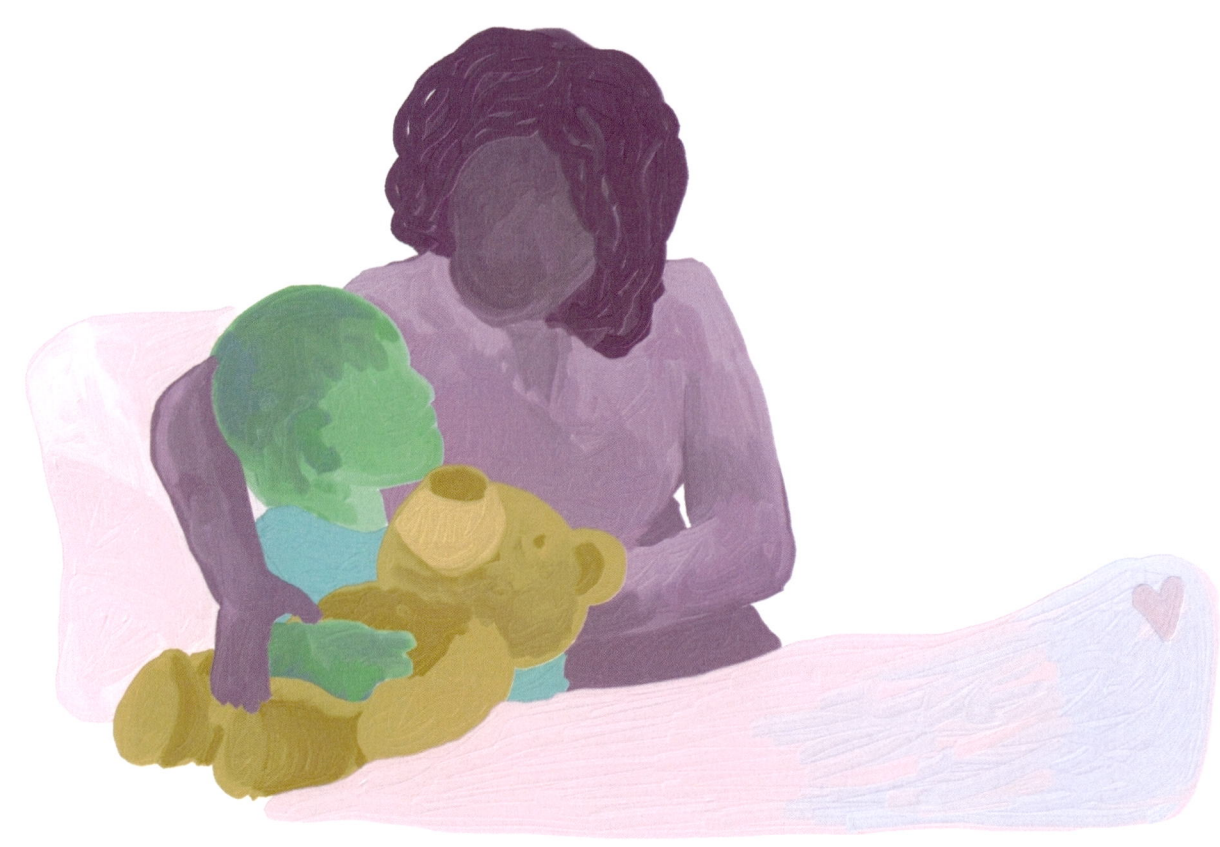

My grown-up talked to the hospital people when I didn't feel like it.
My grown-up snuggled me when I wasn't feeling good.
My grown-up was a great sidekick.

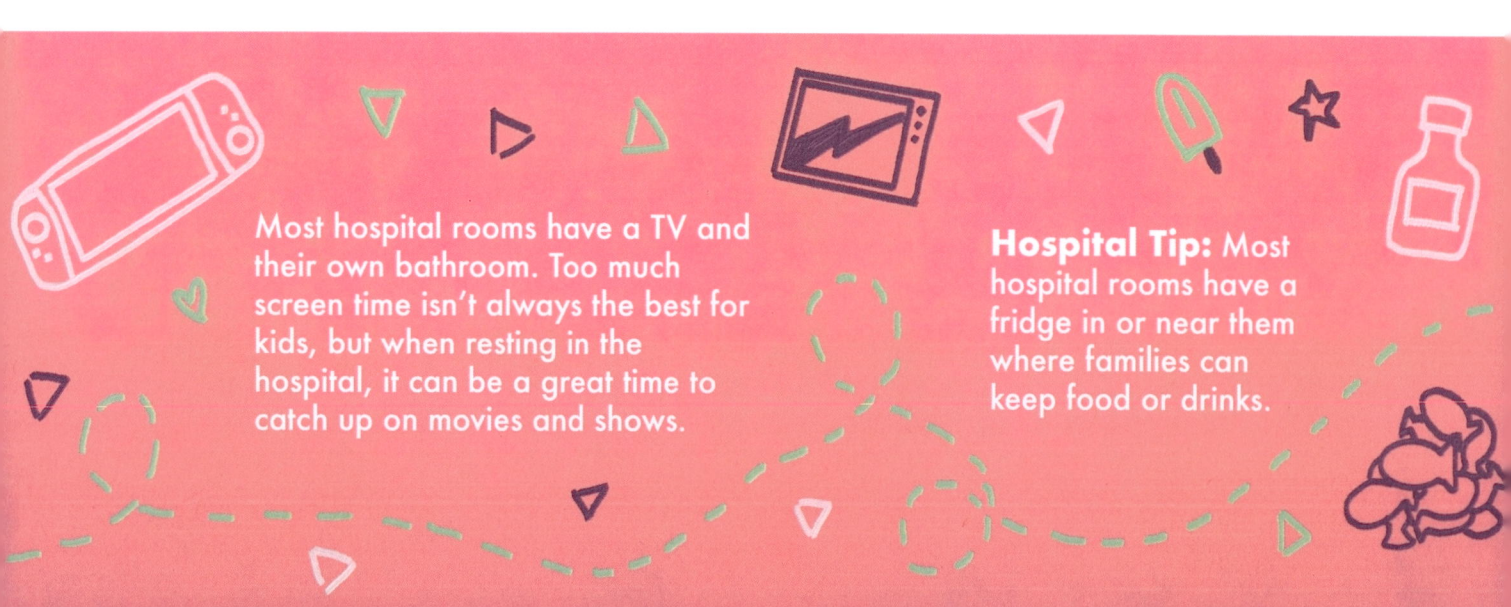

Most hospital rooms have a TV and their own bathroom. Too much screen time isn't always the best for kids, but when resting in the hospital, it can be a great time to catch up on movies and shows.

Hospital Tip: Most hospital rooms have a fridge in or near them where families can keep food or drinks.

Different kids need different things to get better. My doctor and nurse talked to my grown-up and me about different ways that they could help my body.

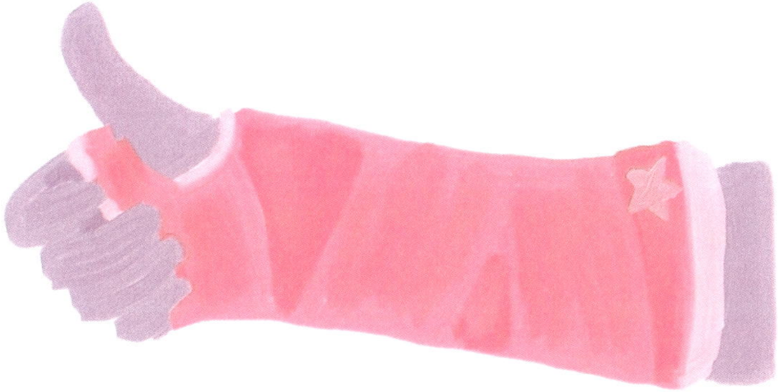

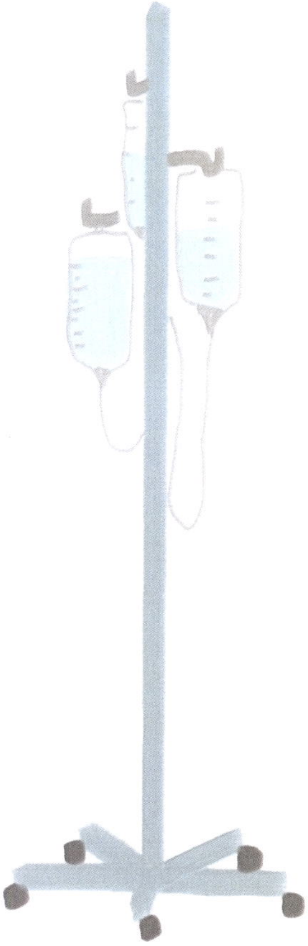

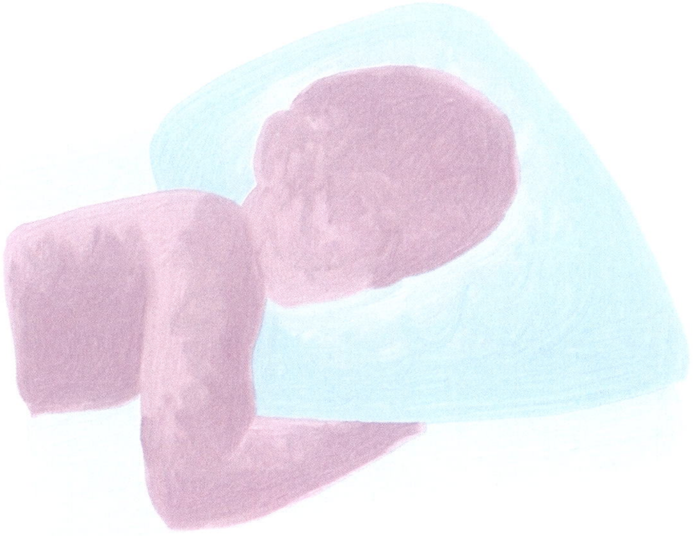

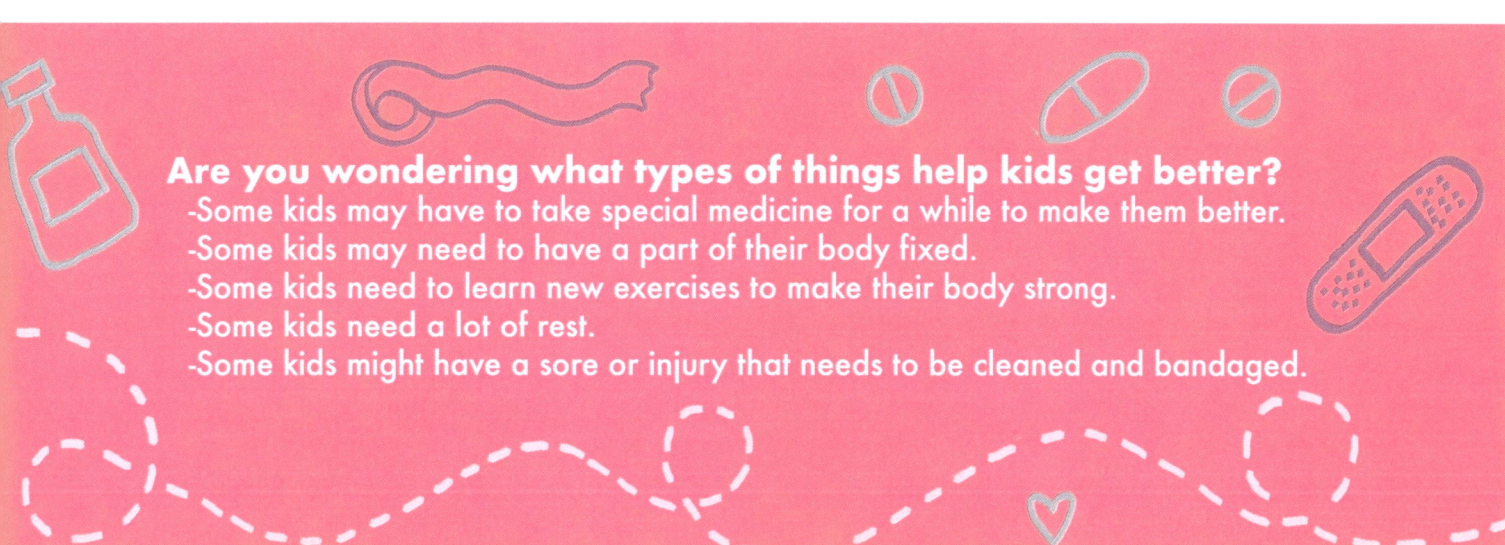

Are you wondering what types of things help kids get better?
-Some kids may have to take special medicine for a while to make them better.
-Some kids may need to have a part of their body fixed.
-Some kids need to learn new exercises to make their body strong.
-Some kids need a lot of rest.
-Some kids might have a sore or injury that needs to be cleaned and bandaged.

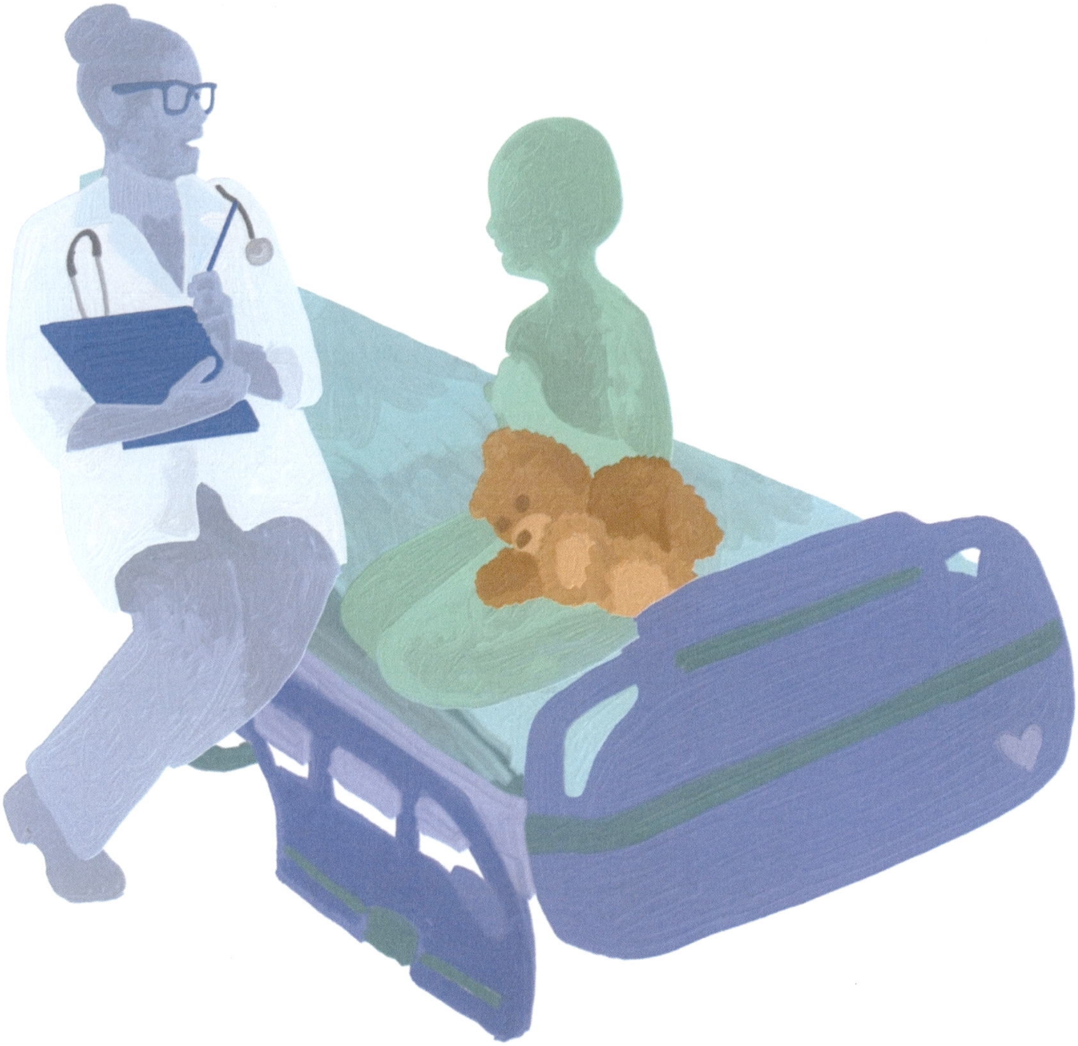

I tried not to worry when I did something new. Instead, I asked questions to learn more. Lots of things weren't as hard as I thought they would be!

When an explorer does new things, it's a good idea for the explorer to try to understand what it will be like and why it's important.

When experiencing something new it can help to ask:

-How long will it last?
-What will I hear, smell, and taste?
-What will it feel like?
-Where will it happen?
-What have other kids done to make it easier?

Check out the 'Ways to Cope' page in the Hospital Adventure Guide for more ideas of how to make hard things easier.

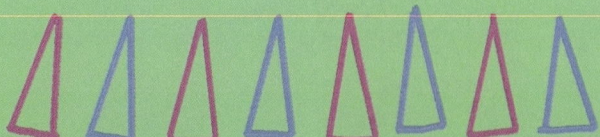

The hospital has its own kitchen called a cafeteria. I got to order food that I liked, and they brought it to my room! Some kids in the hospital have to stop eating for a little while or can only eat certain things while their bodies heal. The nurse helped me know what I could eat.

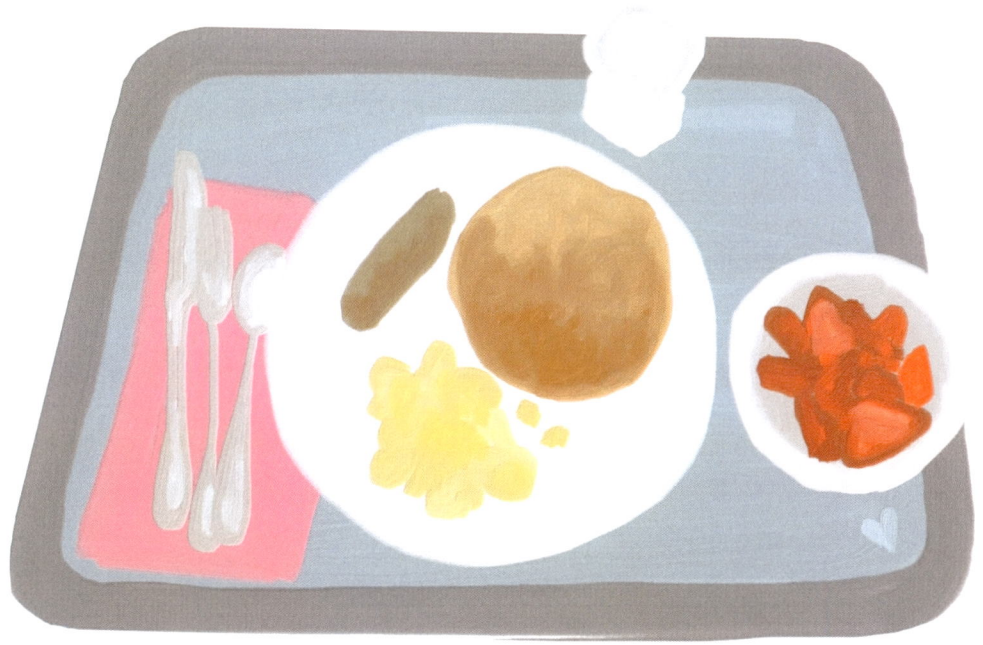

I liked ordering dessert with my food.
Adventures are always better with dessert!

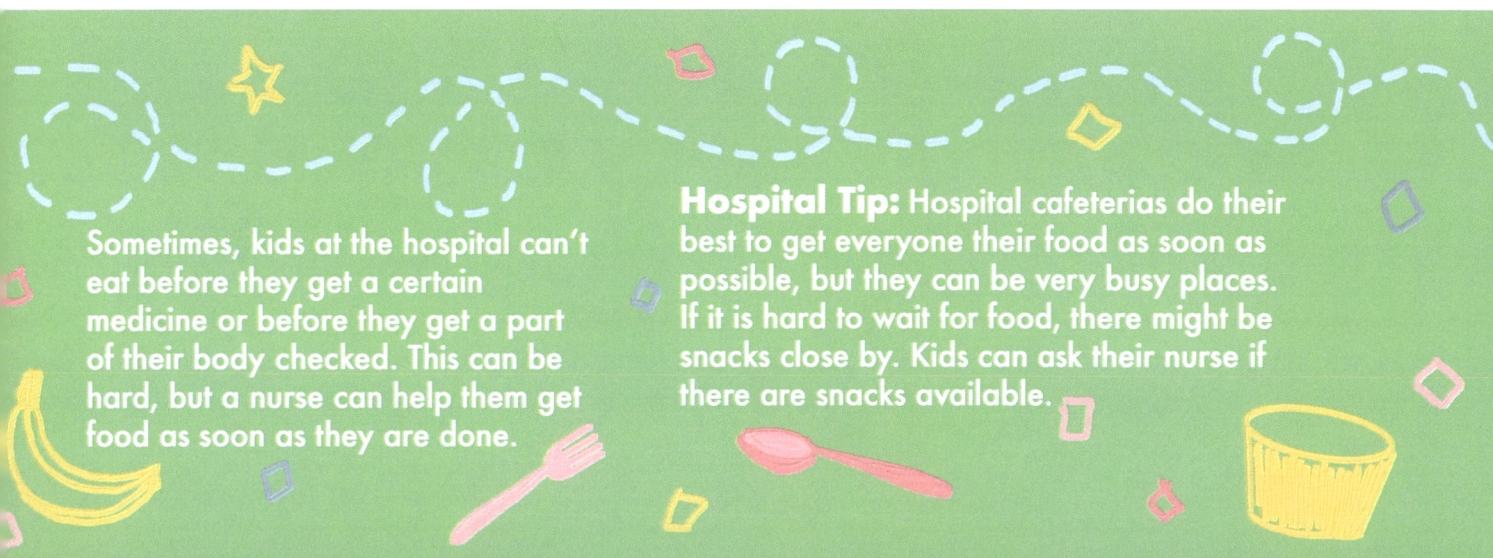

Sometimes, kids at the hospital can't eat before they get a certain medicine or before they get a part of their body checked. This can be hard, but a nurse can help them get food as soon as they are done.

Hospital Tip: Hospital cafeterias do their best to get everyone their food as soon as possible, but they can be very busy places. If it is hard to wait for food, there might be snacks close by. Kids can ask their nurse if there are snacks available.

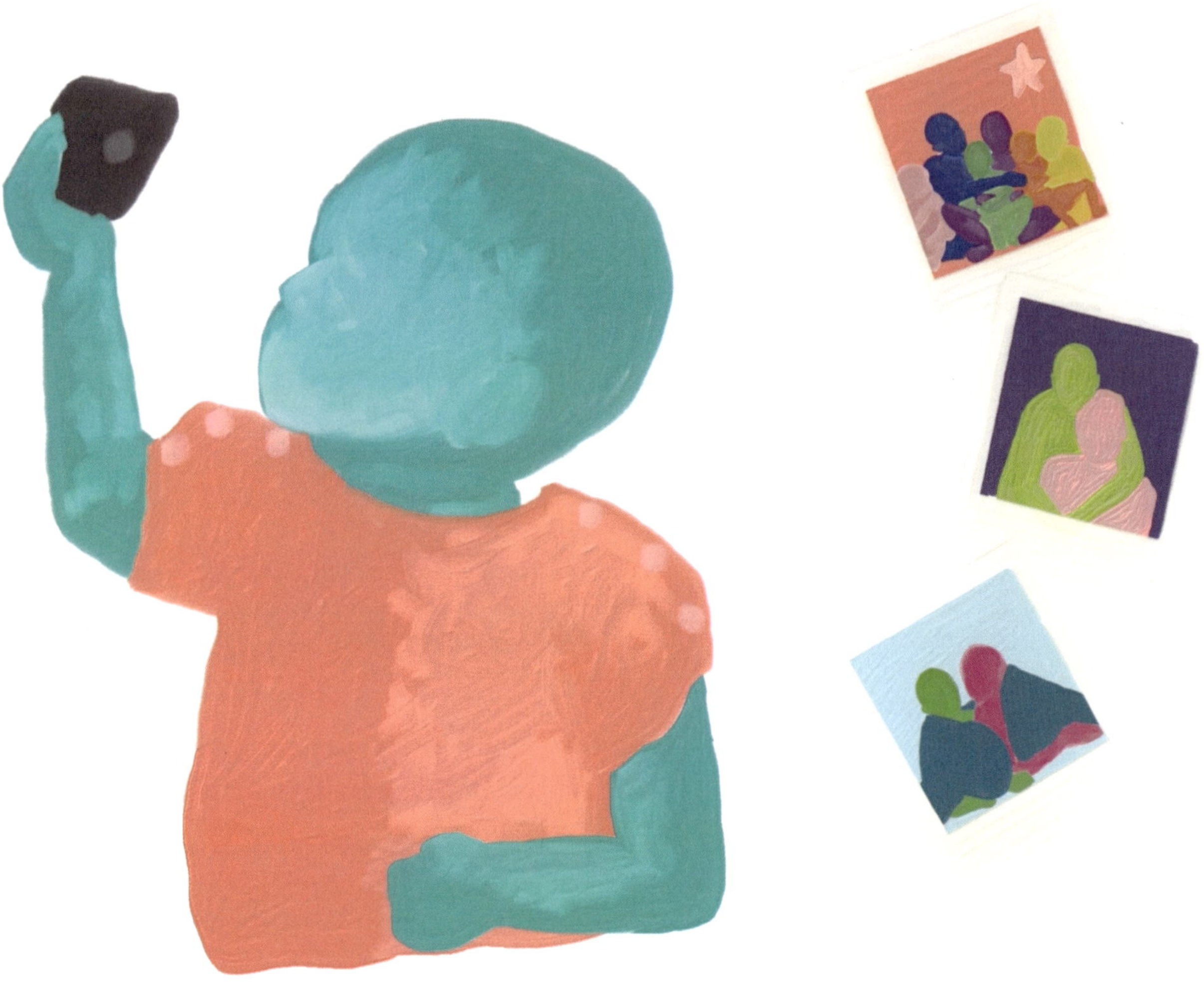

Sometimes, brave explorers start to miss home. When I
would start to miss my family and friends, there were things
that I could do to help. I would talk to the people I missed
on the phone. I would record silly videos and send them.
I really loved seeing the silly videos they sent back!

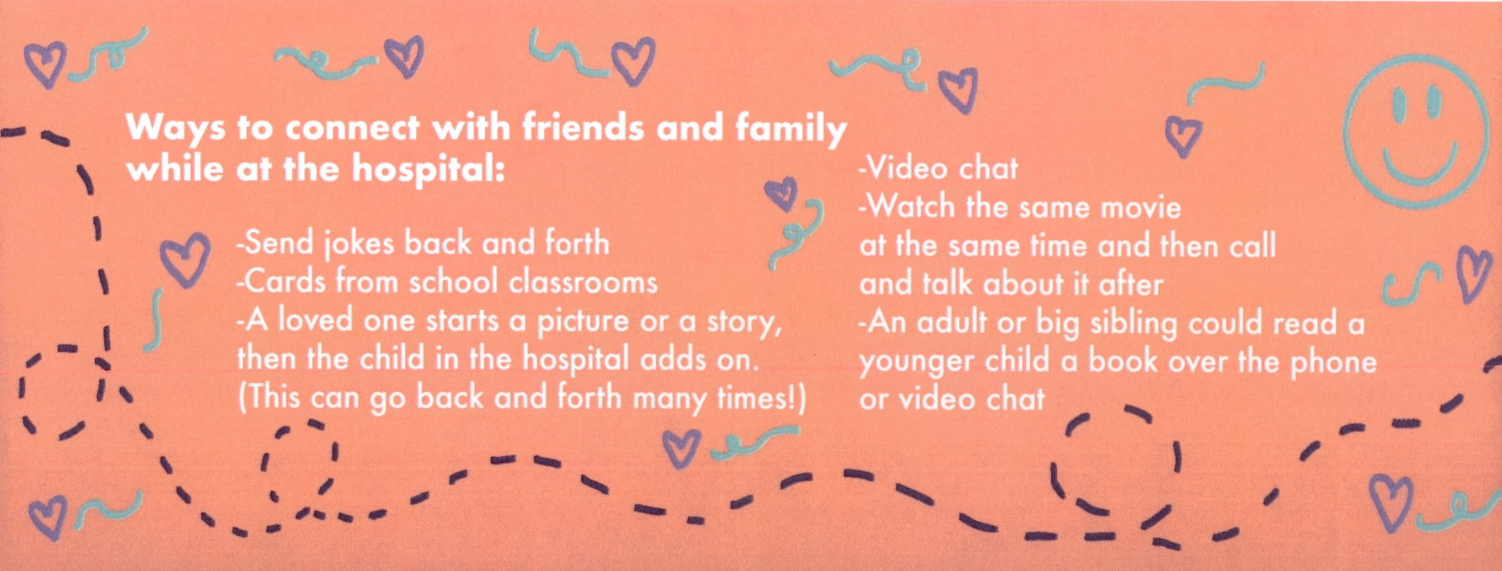

**Ways to connect with friends and family
while at the hospital:**

-Send jokes back and forth
-Cards from school classrooms
-A loved one starts a picture or a story,
then the child in the hospital adds on.
(This can go back and forth many times!)

-Video chat
-Watch the same movie
at the same time and then call
and talk about it after
-An adult or big sibling could read a
younger child a book over the phone
or video chat

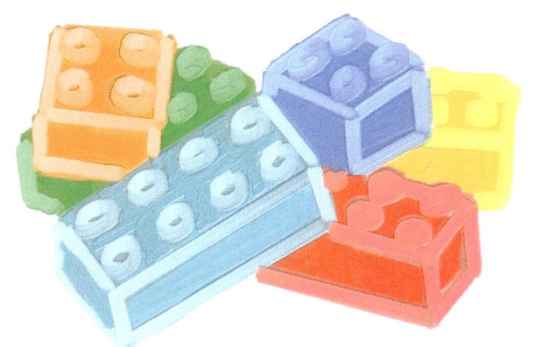

I was so surprised to find out that the hospital had toys! They also told my grown-up that I could bring in my favorite toy from home. So I actually had two sidekicks, my grown-up and my teddy!

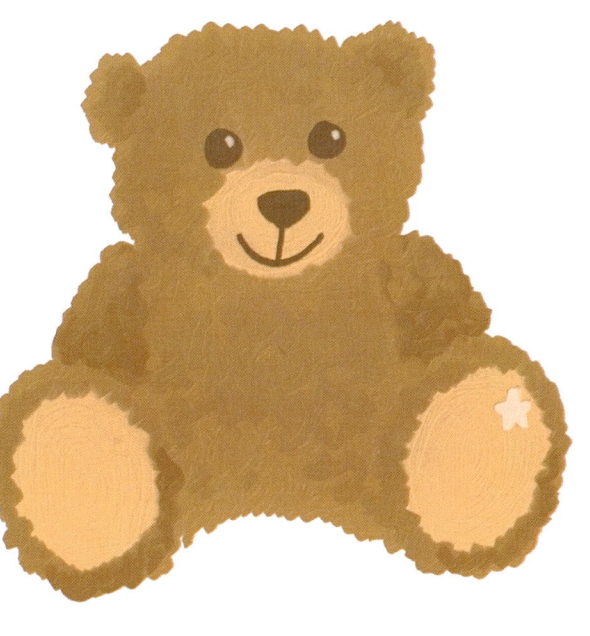

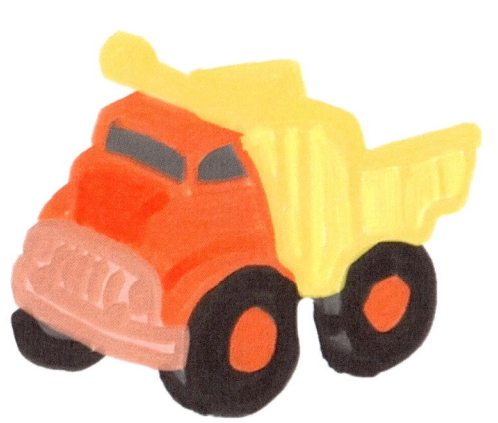

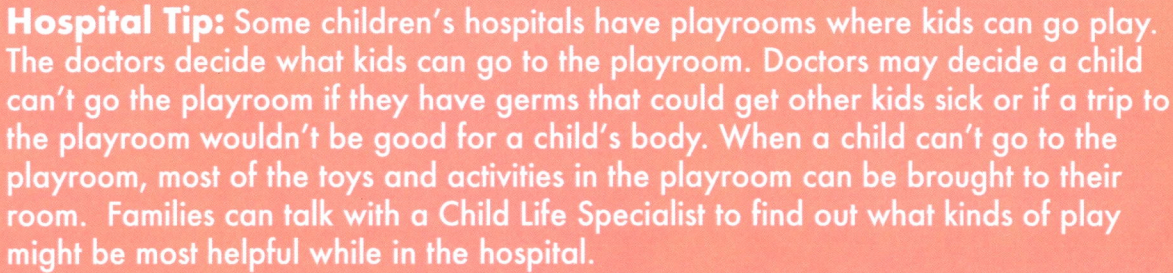

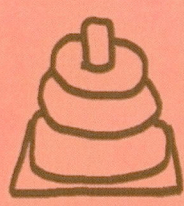

Hospital Tip: Some children's hospitals have playrooms where kids can go play. The doctors decide what kids can go to the playroom. Doctors may decide a child can't go the playroom if they have germs that could get other kids sick or if a trip to the playroom wouldn't be good for a child's body. When a child can't go to the playroom, most of the toys and activities in the playroom can be brought to their room. Families can talk with a Child Life Specialist to find out what kinds of play might be most helpful while in the hospital.

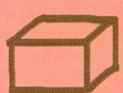
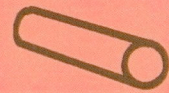

Hospital Tip: Toys and activities get cleaned or thrown away between each child to keep everyone healthy.

When my body didn't need the people and the things at the hospital to get better anymore, I got to go home.
Before I left, the doctors and nurses talked to my grown-up and me about ways to take care of my body at home.

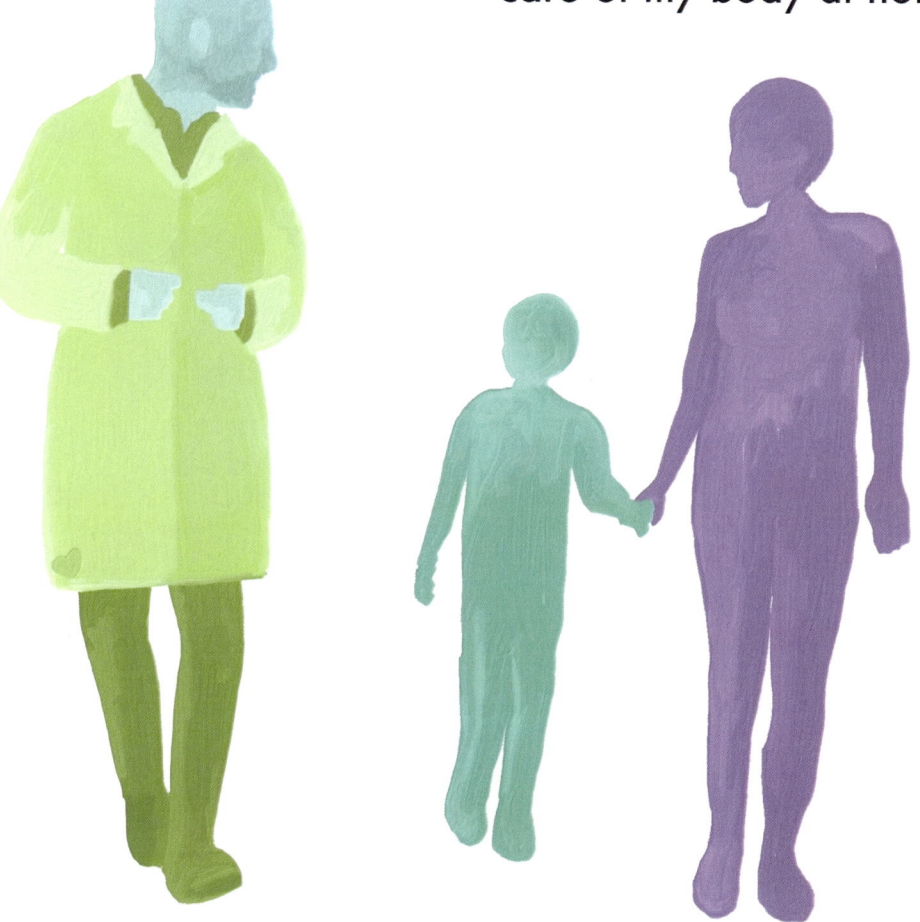

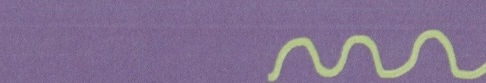

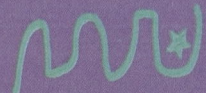

Sometimes, when people come home from the hospital, they still need extra rest. After a hospital stay, you will get instructions about what you can and can't do. It is important to follow these instructions.

Doctors or nurses might suggest things like resting, eating or drinking certain things, taking medicine, or keeping a bandage clean.

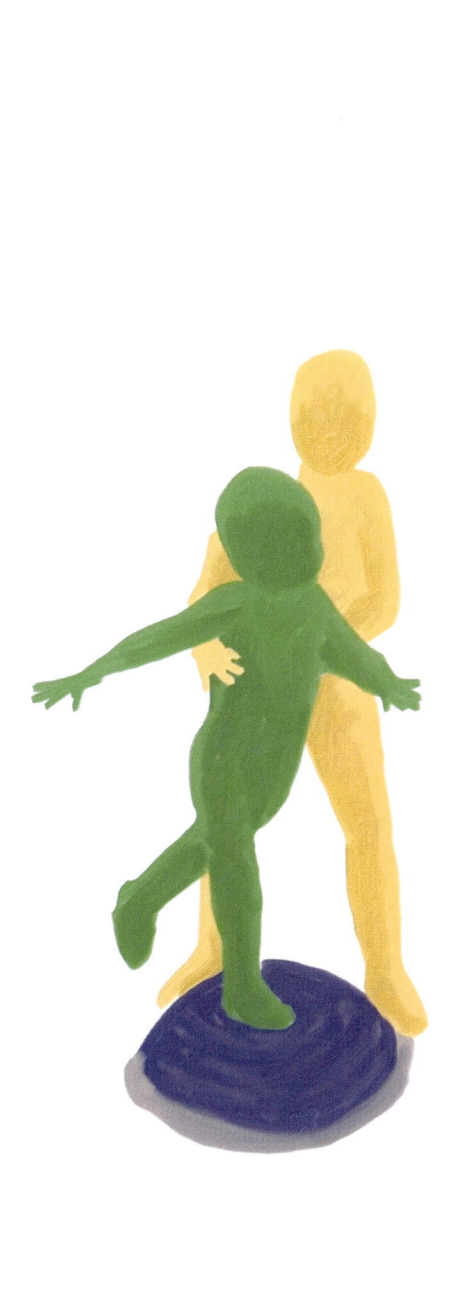

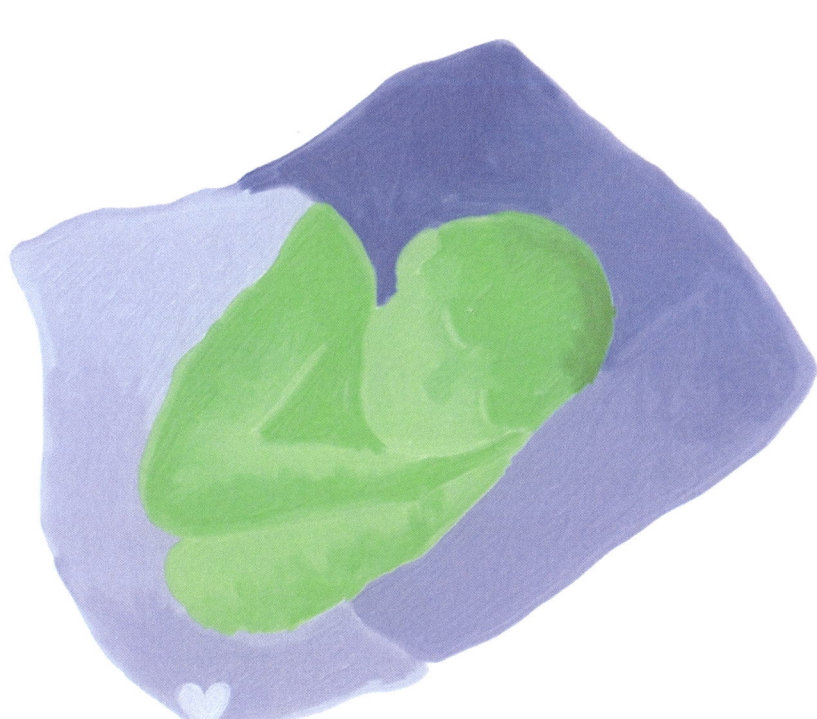

My body needed rest after my hospital adventure. I even learned some exercises that I could do at home to help my body heal. There are lots of things I can do to take care of my body.

When someone comes home from the hospital, they might not be ready for some of their favorite activities. Their family can help them find other fun things to do!

PT/OT: Physical Therapists (PTs) and Occupational Therapists (OTs) work with kids to get their muscles stronger and to teach them new ways to move their bodies. A PT or OT might work with you in the hospital so that you can learn exercises that will help your body.

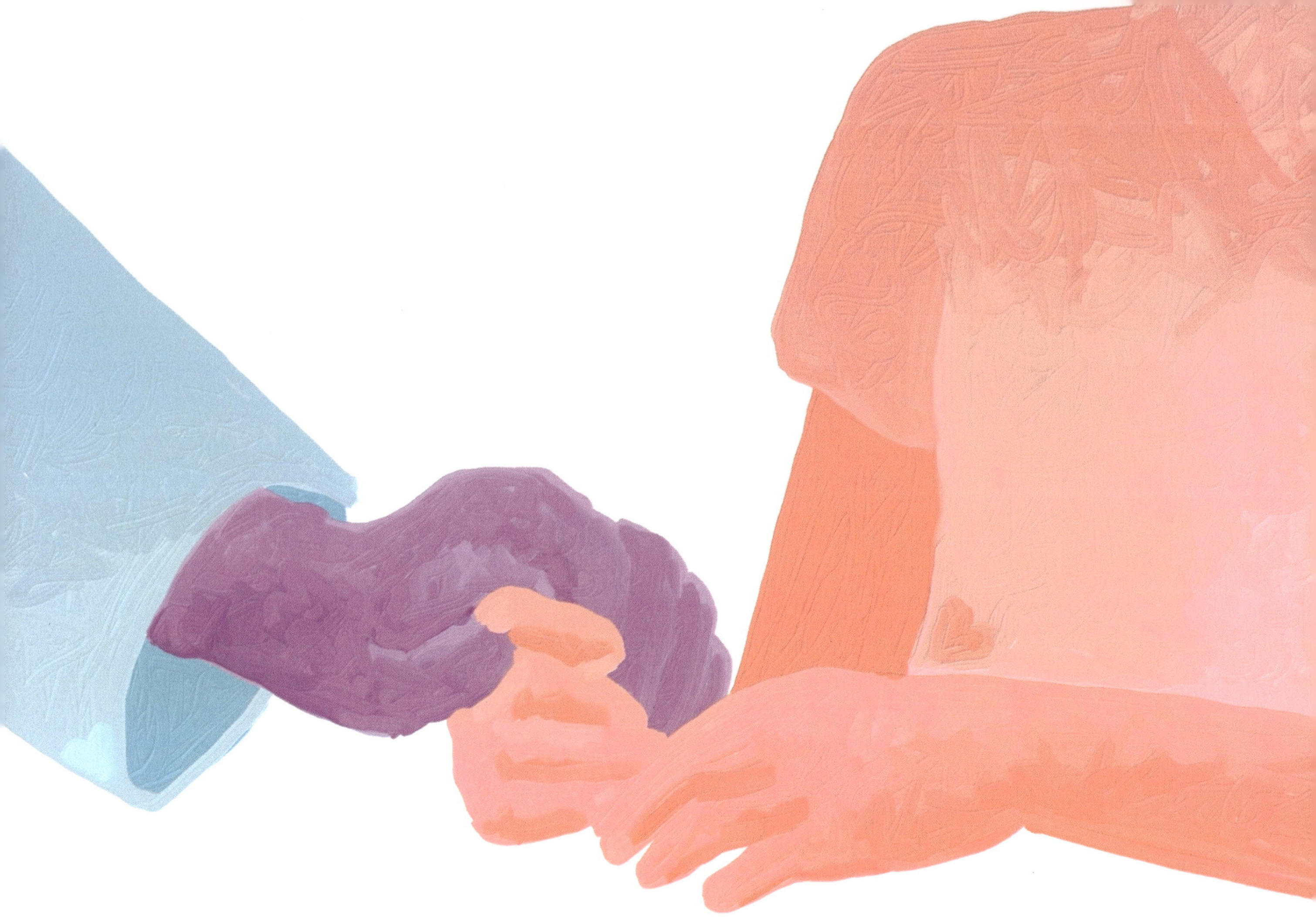

I learned so much on my hospital adventure.
I learned that everyone at the hospital was on my team! They wanted to help me get better so that I could go home.

I am so happy that I had the whole hospital team to help me!

People who work at the hospital don't want you to hurt. They want to help you find ways to be more comfortable. They may use something called a pain scale so that you can tell them how you feel. You can find some new pain scale choices in the Hospital Adventure Guide.

Hospital Tip: If something is hurting or a child is nervous that something will hurt, there are lots of ways that hospitals can help. Options could include numbing creams, pain medicine, breathing exercises, comfortable positions, distractions, and cool/heat packs. Different things work well for different kids and different kinds of pain.

I am a brave hospital explorer!

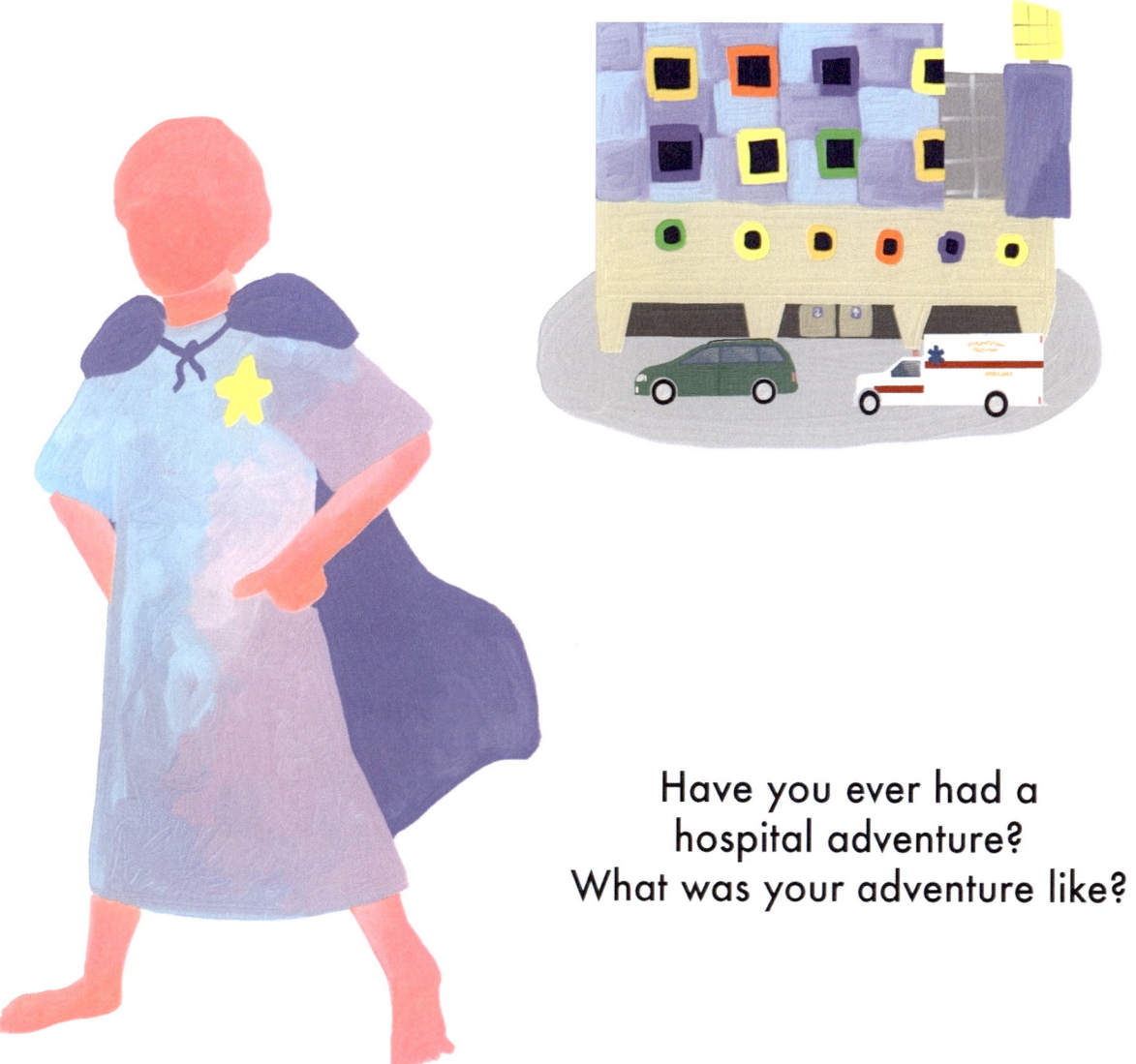

Have you ever had a
hospital adventure?
What was your adventure like?

What do you think the best
part of being in the hospital is?

What do you think the
hardest part is?

You can share your adventure
in the Hospital Adventure
Guide!

Hospital Jokes:

Why did the cookie go to the hospital?
- Because he felt crummy!

Why did the orange go to the hospital?
- She wasn't peeling well!

Where do sick boats go to get healthy?
- To the dock!

Hospital Adventure I Spy:

Go back through the book and see if you can find these things!
Every page has a **heart** and a **star**.
Go back and find them on each page!

You can also find these special hospital items only once in the book:

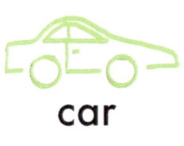 car

banana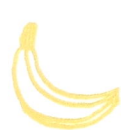

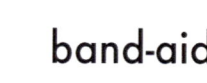 smiley face

band-aid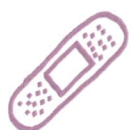

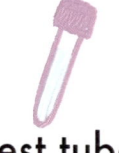 person exercising

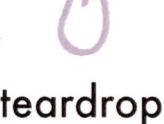 teardrop

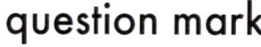 rocket ship

question mark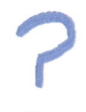

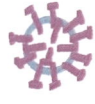 patient bracelet

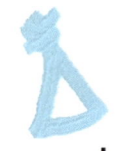 party hat

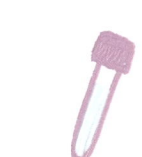 germ

 camera

test tube

ambulance

stethoscope

 tree

 goldfish

cylinder block

moon

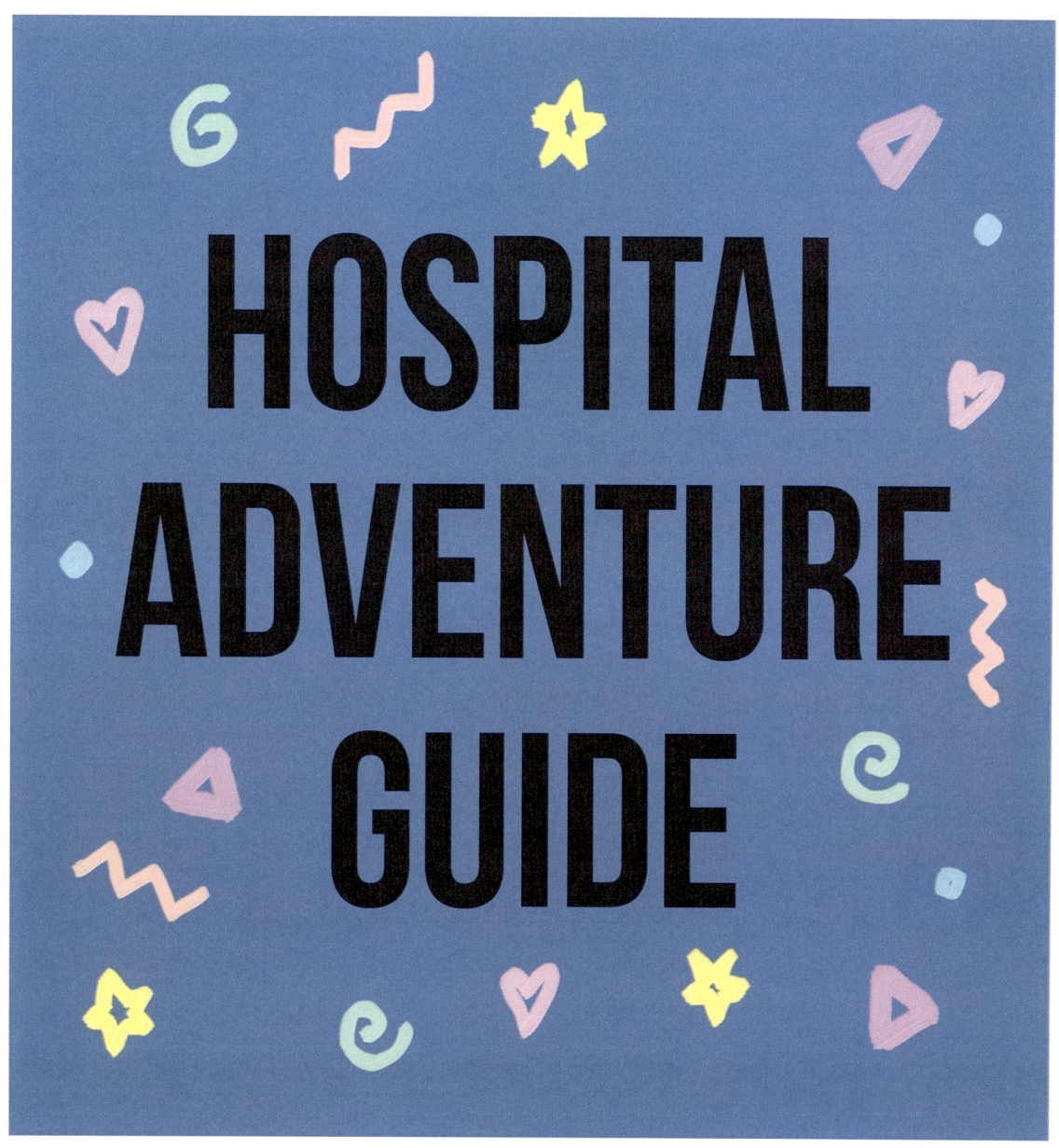

The Hospital Adventure Guide is filled with all sorts of stuff that may be helpful on a hospital adventure. Use it to get more information, and then use the last pages to share your own adventure!

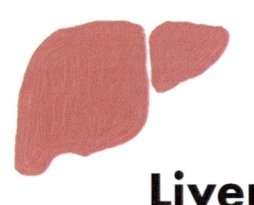

Liver

The liver helps the body use the food and medicine we eat. The liver creates bile to break down the fat in food, and it also helps separate out the things that aren't good for the body.

Gallbladder

The gallbladder stores the bile created by the liver. Bile is used to break down fatty foods.

Pancreas

The pancreas produces enzymes that break down food and insulin, which controls the amount of sugar in a person's blood.

Appendix

The appendix is a small pouch that contains good bacteria that help people feel better after they are sick. Sometimes, the appendix gets blocked or filled with bad bacteria, and it needs to be removed.

Kidneys and Bladder

The kidneys help the blood keep healthy amounts of salt and minerals. They also remove extra liquid from our body and move it into the bladder so that it can be peed out.

Esophagus

The espophagus connects the mouth and the stomach. Its muscles move the food a person eats downward and keeps stomach juices from going up.

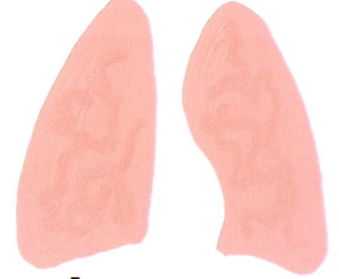

Lungs

The lungs breathe air in and out. When air comes in, the lungs take the oxygen from the air and put it into the blood. The lungs also take the carbon dioxide out of the blood and help the body breathe it out.

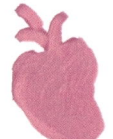

Heart

The heart is connected to tiny tubes called veins and arteries. They carry the blood around our body. The heart pumps the blood and keeps it moving through these tubes. The blood carries oxygen and other important things to every part of the body.

Stomach

The stomach holds the food and mixes it with acid. The acid breaks down the food so that the body can use it.

Intestines

The intestines are a long tube that food travels through after leaving the stomach. Enzymes in the intestines break down food more, keeping the good things for the body to use and forming the rest into poop.

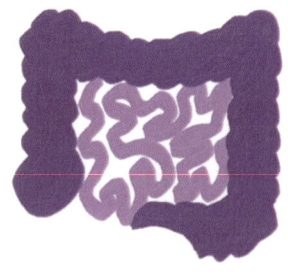

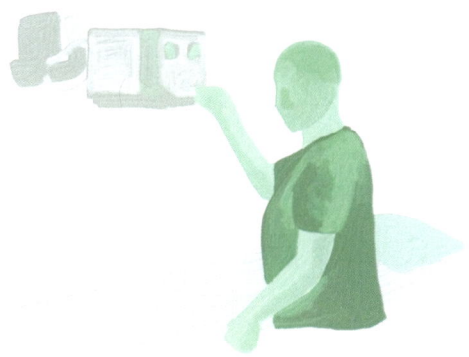

X-Ray: Line up this camera with a light, then a quick picture, and it's done. Many doctors use x-rays to look for broken bones or sick lungs.

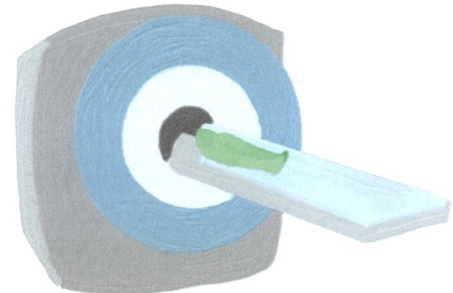

MRI & CT: An MRI and a CT are two different kinds of cameras. Both of them look like big donuts! The person lies on a bed that slides inside the donut. The donut does not touch the person. In order to get a good picture, the person has to hold really still. For a CT, it takes a couple of minutes. For a MRI, it takes longer. MRIs can also be noisy. There are ear plugs or headphones to help.

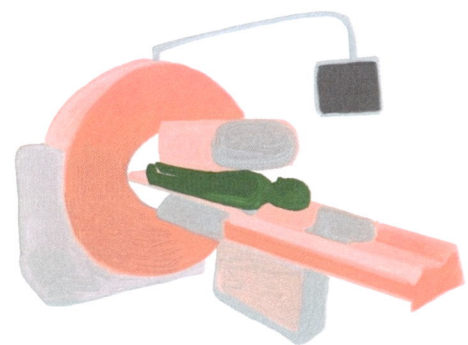

Nuclear Medicine: This camera takes pictures of something called a tracer to see where it goes in the body. The person is given something to eat with the tracer inside or the tracer is put in through an IV. This kind of picture takes a little longer, but still doesn't hurt.

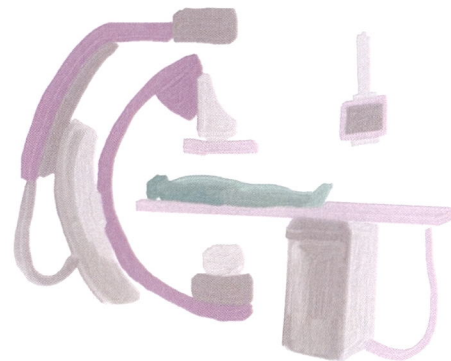

Fluoroscopy: An x-ray video! It doesn't just take a picture. It shows movement. Fluoroscopy cameras can be different shapes. The doctor can see the x-ray video on the computer screen in the room.

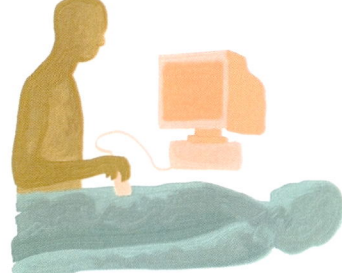

Ultrasound: This camera takes pictures with a device called a wand. The wand is covered with a warm, clear gel so that it slides over the skin. The wand does not hurt, but it does take pictures of what is going on underneath the skin and sends them to a computer.

Ways to Cope With New or Hard Things

Different things help different kids. Read below to get some ideas of what could help you. Talk to the people at your hospital to learn more about what you could try.

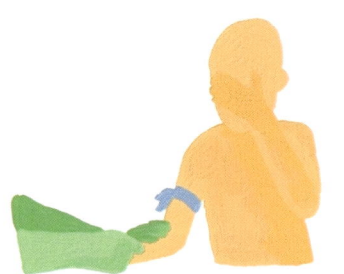

Making Choices:
You and your family know you the best. Think about what has worked well for you in the past. Here are some choices that help some kids:

Do you want to watch or look away?
Remember that you will need to be able to hold your body still.

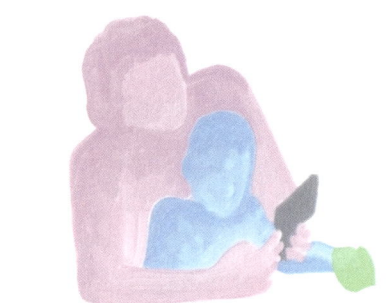

Do you want to try to think about something else?
Many kids find that it is helpful to focus on something else like a tablet/phone, an ISpy book, remembering your favorite trip/place, or even having your grown-up sing your favorite song or quiz you on math facts.

Who do you want to be with you?
Many times it is okay for your grown-up to be with you. Sometimes, they can sit right next to you or hold your hand.

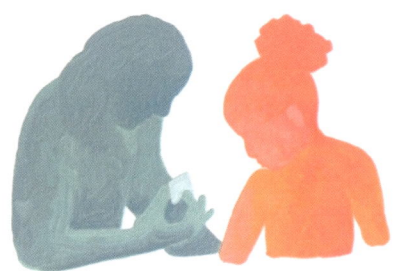

Do you want to know all the details?
For some kids, it helps to know exactly what will happen and how it will feel, smell, and look. For some kids, thinking about the details will make them more nervous. They may just want to be talked through it as it happens.

Breathing Exercises:
When your body and brain get nervous or worried, you can feel like you don't have control. Your body wants to run away or fight, but neither of those options will help you in the hospital. By taking deep breaths, you can calm your body and take control. Then you can make choices that will actually help.

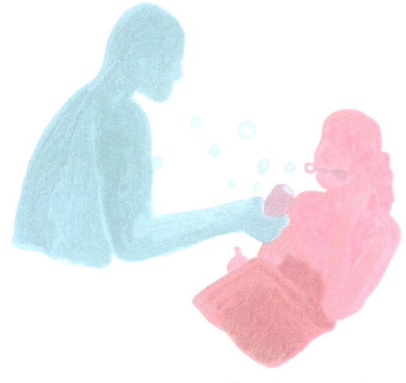

Bubble Blowing: Blowing bubbles is a good way to turn deep breaths into play. This can help you think about something good while also taking deep breaths. You can also try blowing a feather or the hair of a doll to see it move.

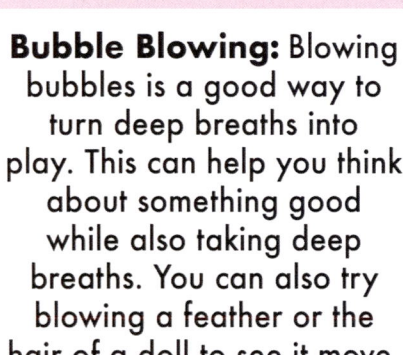

Starfish Breaths: Take a finger and trace your other hand. Breathe in through your nose, as your finger traces up a finger, and out through your mouth, as your finger traces down a finger. Match your movement with your breath.

Ocean Breaths: Breathe in through your nose and then cover your ears and exhale with a "shhh" sound.

Belly Breaths: Put your hands on your belly. Take in a slow breath through your nose and out through your mouth feeling your belly rise and fall.

Pain Scales

Each person experiences pain a little differently. Some things that help one person don't help the next person very much. While at the hospital, a person might try a few different things before they find what works best for them. Doctors and nurses will suggest what has worked for other people. Some things that help with pain can take a while to start working. You can try distracting yourself or use some of the breathing techniques on page 4 while you are waiting for pain medicine to start working.

People at the hospital might ask you to rate your pain. People at the hospital don't want you to hurt, and so this is how they can check to see if the pain is getting better or worse.

Depending on your age and how you think, different pain scales might make more sense for you. You can choose from the scales below. Once you start with one scale, it is usually best to keep using that same one.

1 2 3 4 5 6 7 8 9 10

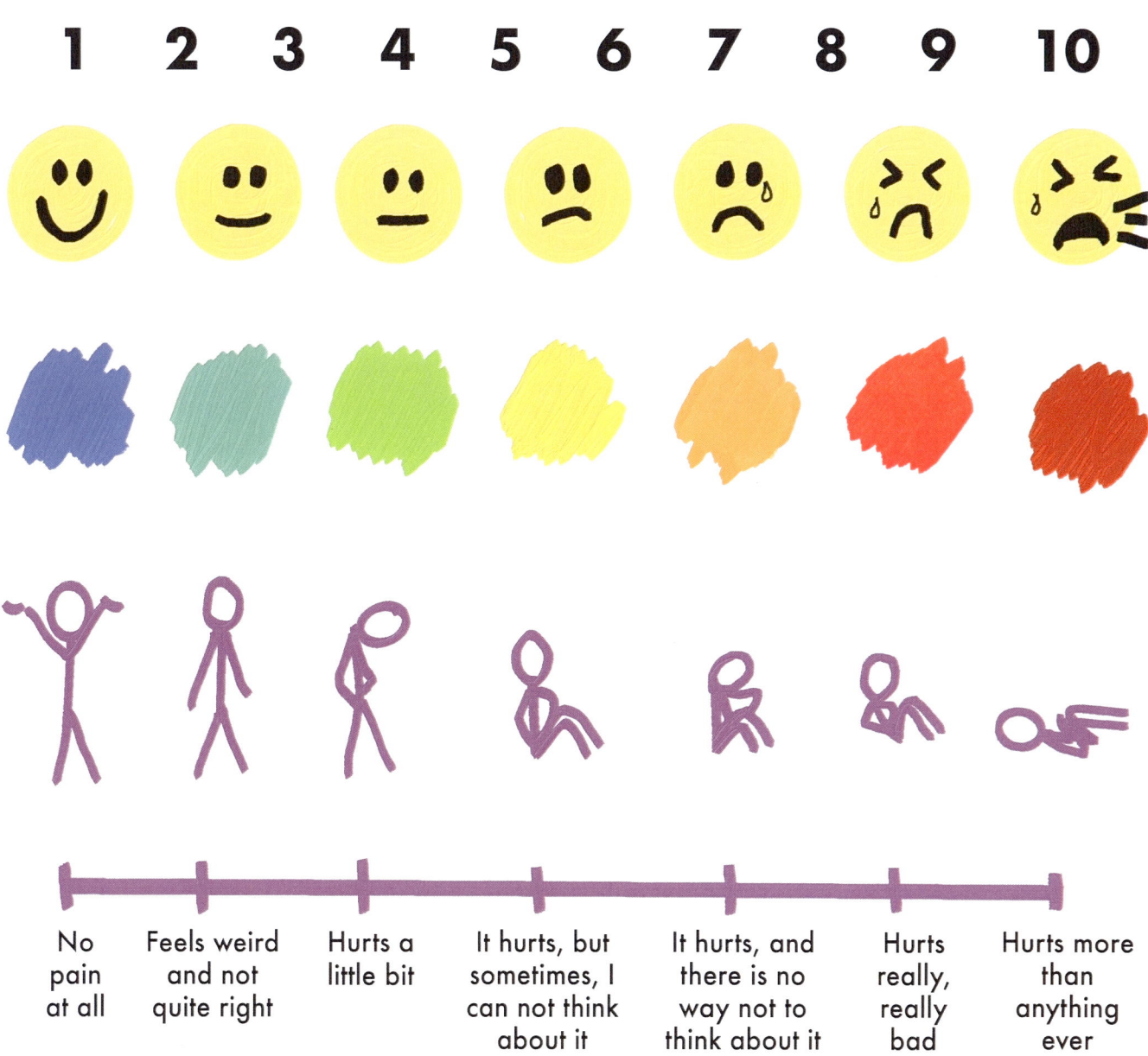

| No pain at all | Feels weird and not quite right | Hurts a little bit | It hurts, but sometimes, I can not think about it | It hurts, and there is no way not to think about it | Hurts really, really bad | Hurts more than anything ever |

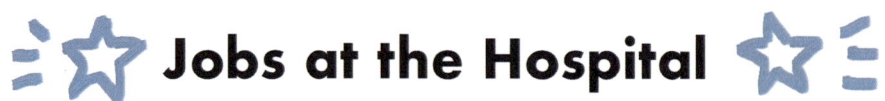

Jobs at the Hospital

Checklist & Place to Record Names (or Answers to Silly Questions)

- [ ] Doctor - Hospitalist - - - - - - - - - - - - - - - - - - - _____
- [ ] Doctor - Specialist - _____
- [ ] Resident Doctor - _____
- [ ] Nurse - _____
- [ ] Housekeeper - _____
- [ ] Patient Transport - _____
- [ ] Food Service - _____
- [ ] Nursing Assistant (CNA) - - - - - - - - - - - - - - - _____
- [ ] Patient Care Tech - _____
- [ ] Unit Clerk - _____
- [ ] Phlebotomist - _____
- [ ] X-Ray Tech - _____
- [ ] Child Life Specialist - - - - - - - - - - - - - - - - - - _____
- [ ] Music Therapist - _____
- [ ] Social Worker - _____
- [ ] Interpreter - _____
- [ ] Dietician - _____
- [ ] Physical Therapist (PT) - - - - - - - - - - - - - - - - _____
- [ ] Occupational Therapist (OT) - - - - - - - - - - - - _____
- [ ] Speech Language Pathologist (SLP) - - - - - - - _____
- [ ] Transport Nurse (helicopter nurse) - - - - - - - - _____
- [ ] Therapist - _____
- [ ] Student (medical, nursing, radiology, etc.) - - _____
- [ ] Teacher - _____
- [ ] Chaplain - _____
- [ ] Volunteer - _____

My Hospital Advenure

Why did you need to go to the hospital? _____

_____

My favorite people at the hospital are: _____

_____

The hardest part of my adventure was: _____

_____

My favorite part of the adventure was: _____

_____

The best hospital food was: _____

If I knew someone else going on a hospital adventure, I would tell
them: _____

_____

A Picture of Me in the Hospital

_____'S HOSPITAL ADVENTURE

CREATE A SILLY EXCITING ADVENTURE ABOUT YOU OR ANOTHER CHARACTER!

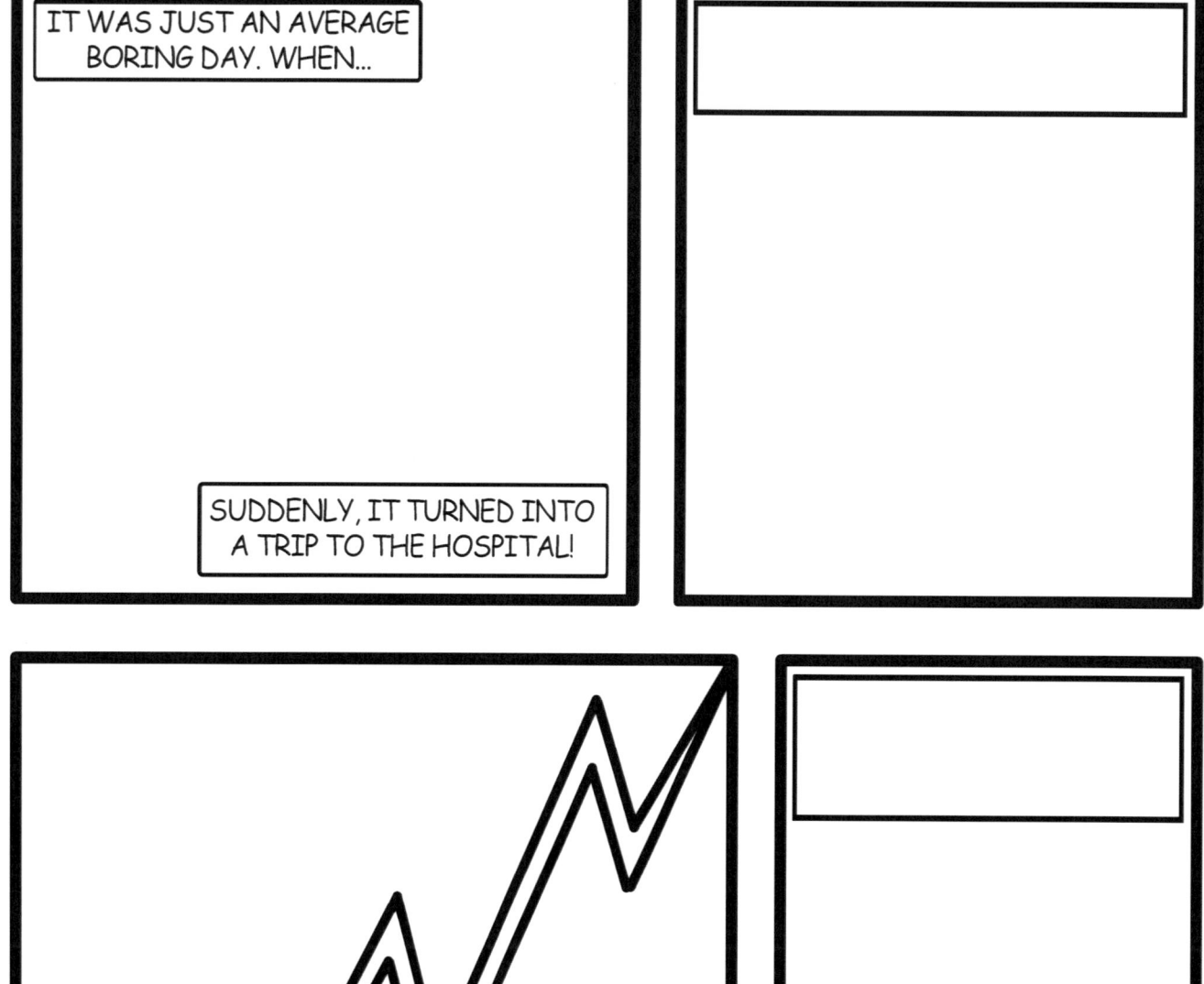

IT WAS JUST AN AVERAGE BORING DAY. WHEN...

SUDDENLY, IT TURNED INTO A TRIP TO THE HOSPITAL!

THE END!

YOU CAN SHARE YOUR HOSPITAL STORY OR COMIC WITH THE WORLD.
TAKE A PICTURE AND HAVE AN ADULT SHARE IT ON INSTAGRAM.
TAG @WORDS.WORTH.REPEATING!

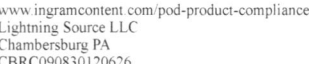